THE
EVERYTHING®
GUIDE TO MANAGING
TYPE 2 DIABETES

Dear Reader,

Diabetes can be a scary and confusing disease. This is especially true at diagnosis, when all you may know about the condition is that (a) there is no cure and (b) there are needles and daily blood tests involved.

It isn't just the diabetes that frightens us—it's also the host of long-term complications, emotional baggage, and lifestyle challenges that are packaged with the disease. There are many "unknowns" with diabetes.

Whether you're newly diagnosed with diabetes or are a diabetes veteran, gaining knowledge of the disease is your best tool for achieving a healthier and happier life. And that's where *The Everything® Guide to Managing Type 2 Diabetes* comes in.

This book is also a guide for the millions of caregivers—spouses, parents, adult children, and others—who live with or care for someone who has diabetes. The support you give your loved one is crucial to his or her long-term wellness.

Balancing blood sugars day in and day out is a difficult and sometimes frustrating experience. The good news is that with information and good care, such a balance *is* achievable. *The Everything® Guide to Managing Type 2 Diabetes* teaches you how to control your diabetes, and not to let it control you.

Paula Ford-Martin

Welcome to the EVERYTHING® Series!

These handy, accessible books give you all you need to tackle a difficult project, gain a new hobby, comprehend a fascinating topic, prepare for an exam, or even brush up on something you learned back in school but have since forgotten.

You can choose to read an Everything® book from cover to cover or just pick out the information you want from our four useful boxes: e-questions, e-facts, e-alerts, and e-ssentials.

We give you everything you need to know on the subject, but throw in a lot of fun stuff along the way, too.

We now have more than 400 Everything® books in print, spanning such wide-ranging categories as weddings, pregnancy, cooking, music instruction, foreign language, crafts, pets, New Age, and so much more. When you're done reading them all, you can finally say you know Everything®!

QUESTION

Answers to
common questions

FACT

Important snippets
of information

ALERT

Urgent
warnings

ESSENTIAL

Quick
handy tips

PUBLISHER Karen Cooper

MANAGING EDITOR, EVERYTHING® SERIES Lisa Laing

COPY CHIEF Casey Ebert

ASSOCIATE PRODUCTION EDITOR Mary Beth Dolan

ACQUISITIONS EDITOR Brett Palana-Shanahan

SENIOR DEVELOPMENT EDITOR Brett Palana-Shanahan

EVERYTHING® SERIES COVER DESIGNER Erin Alexander

Visit the entire Everything® series at *www.everything.com*

THE
EVERYTHING®
GUIDE TO MANAGING TYPE 2 DIABETES

From diagnosis to diet, all you need to live a healthy,
active life with type 2 diabetes

Paula Ford-Martin with Jason Baker, MD

Adams Media
New York London Toronto Sydney New Delhi

For all my editorial homegirls. Zen, Monica, Kerri, Lynn, Kate, Erin, and Julia—your hearts, smarts, and kindness will always inspire me.

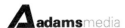

Adams Media
An Imprint of Simon & Schuster, Inc.
57 Littlefield Street
Avon, Massachusetts 02322

Copyright © 2013 by Simon & Schuster, Inc.

An Everything® Series Book.

Everything® and everything.com® are registered trademarks of Simon & Schuster, Inc.

ADAMS MEDIA and colophon are trademarks of Simon and Schuster.

For information about special discounts for bulk purchases, please contact Simon & Schuster Special Sales at 1-866-506-1949 or business@simonandschuster.com.

The Simon & Schuster Speakers Bureau can bring authors to your live event. For more information or to book an event contact the Simon & Schuster Speakers Bureau at 1-866-248-3049 or visit our website at www.simonspeakers.com.

Manufactured in the United States of America

10 9 8 7

Library of Congress Cataloging-in-Publication Data has been applied for.

ISBN 978-1-4405-5196-3
ISBN 978-1-4405-5197-0 (ebook)

This book is intended as general information only, and should not be used to diagnose or treat any health condition. In light of the complex, individual, and specific nature of health problems, this book is not intended to replace professional medical advice. The ideas, procedures, and suggestions in this book are intended to supplement, not replace, the advice of a trained medical professional. Consult your physician before adopting any of the suggestions in this book, as well as about any condition that may require diagnosis or medical attention. The author and publisher disclaim any liability arising directly or indirectly from the use of this book.

This publication is designed to provide accurate and authoritative information with regard to the subject matter covered. It is sold with the understanding that the publisher is not engaged in rendering legal, accounting, or other professional advice. If legal advice or other expert assistance is required, the services of a competent professional person should be sought.

—From a *Declaration of Principles* jointly adopted by a Committee of the American Bar Association and a Committee of Publishers and Associations

Contents

Acknowledgments

I would not have been able to finish this book, in record time, without the support and encouragement of my wonderful husband, Tim. I'd also like to thank my kids—Cassie, Kate, Chris, and John—for the silence, self-sufficiency, and occasional "how's it goin'?" so I could keep my head down all the way to the finish line. Thanks to Barb Doyen, my agent, for crossing t's and dotting i's in her usual expedient and helpful manner; to Dr. Jason Baker for his thoughtful clinical review; and to Brett Shanahan, my editor, for getting this project approved and moving it forward.

Introduction

IF YOU'VE PICKED UP this book, chances are that type 2 diabetes has touched your life or the life of someone close to you. Diabetes can be a frightening and personally devastating diagnosis. Fortunately, learning all you can about diabetes and seeking support are probably the two most important components to staying on top of this disease.

A key phrase in the lexicon of diabetes care is good control. For those of you who are new to diabetes, good control means keeping your blood glucose, or blood sugar, in a range at or close to normal through diet, exercise, and/or medication (which can include pills, insulin, and/or other injectable drugs). Control is the answer to the physical and emotional management of diabetes. Always remember that the power is in your hands to determine how diabetes affects your life.

Unfortunately, many people feel out of control of their diabetes. Some ignore it completely in a fog of denial. Others follow medical instructions to the letter, yet never ask questions of their doctors nor provide any feedback to them. The latter group may get a handle on their blood sugar levels, but are so miserable it hardly matters.

Managing diabetes requires knowledge, dedication, and a certain doggedness of character. Most importantly, it requires a commitment to being a leader, not a follower, in terms of your own health care. Surrounding yourself with good people—endocrinologists and diabetologists, certified diabetes educators, registered dietitians, and others—is an excellent start to effectively managing diabetes. But it takes more than a crack medical team to control diabetes. Playing an active role in your own health care—as coach of your health care team—is essential for staying both healthy and happy. So is surrounding yourself with people who care about you and are willing to support you in your pursuit of wellness.

High blood sugar levels can affect every system of the body over time if not managed properly. Heart disease, stroke, vision loss, kidney disease, and nerve damage are just a few of the complications that uncontrolled diabetes leaves in its wake. This is why educating yourself about good diabetes management—through diet, exercise, medication, lifestyle, and more—is so very essential.

Medical breakthroughs, such as continuous glucose monitoring technologies, new oral and injectable medications and insulin formulations, insulin pumps, and others have drastically improved the quality of life for all people with diabetes. But until there is a cure for this disease, staying current on developments in diabetes management, communicating with your health care team, and staying on top of self care through healthy lifestyle choices are absolutely essential to wellness. *The Everything® Guide to Managing Type 2 Diabetes* was designed to be your reference partner in staying healthy with diabetes.

CHAPTER 1

What Is Diabetes?

Diabetes mellitus comes in many varieties—type 1, type 2, gestational, and variations such as maturity-onset diabetes of the young (MODY) and latent autoimmune diabetes in adults (LADA). Regardless of the name, people with diabetes share a common trait: Their bodies have an inherent inability to self-regulate the levels of blood glucose—or cellular fuel. In particular, type 2 diabetes accounts for 90 to 95 percent of U.S. diabetes cases and is one of the most serious and fastest growing health threats to Americans.

A Growing Problem

The U.S. Centers for Disease Control and Prevention (CDC) has called diabetes "an emerging epidemic." The statistics say it all. As of 2011, the CDC put the number of U.S. residents living with diabetes at a staggering 25.8 million people, of which 7 million of these individuals don't even know they have the disease. In other words, 8.3 percent of the entire U.S. population is living with diabetes. And another 79 million Americans over age twenty (35 percent of the population) have prediabetes, a condition that is a precursor to type 2 diabetes. Many lack important knowledge of the condition and the consequences.

FACT

Type 2 diabetes accounts for 90 to 95 percent of the total diabetes population in the United States and is the seventh leading cause of death in America. But moderate levels of regular physical activity and a healthy diet can cut a person's chance of developing type 2 by 58 to 71 percent.

In addition to the physical and emotional toll it exacts, diabetes also comes with an enormous price tag. An American living with diabetes has health care costs that are three times higher than those without the disease. According to the American Diabetes Association (ADA), the disease costs Americans $174 billion annually in medical expenses and lost productivity. And it isn't just diabetes that's running up the tab. Nearly $58 billion of those costs were for direct expenses related to chronic diabetic complications, which translates to a cost of approximately $11,774 per patient.

The Endocrine System

Diabetes mellitus is a disease of the endocrine system. The endocrine system is composed of glands that secrete the hormones that travel through the circulatory and lymph systems. These hormones regulate metabolism, growth, sexual development, and reproduction. When one of these glands—the adrenals, the thyroid and parathyroids, the thymus, the pituitary, testes, ovaries, and the pancreas—secretes either too little or too much of a hormone, the entire body can be thrown off balance.

ESSENTIAL

While the term *diabetic* is a useful adjective for describing things and conditions related to diabetes—diabetic supplies, diabetic kidney disease, and so on—some people with the disease bristle at being labeled "a diabetic." People with diabetes should not have to be defined by the disease, nor be marginalized because of it.

The Pancreas and Liver

One of the endocrine glands—the pancreas—actually pulls double duty as a digestive organ. Sitting behind the stomach, the spongy pancreas secretes both digestive enzymes and endocrine hormones. It is long and tapered with a thicker bottom end (or head), which is cradled in the downward curve of the duodenum—the first portion of the small intestine or bowel. The long end (or tail) of the pancreas extends up behind the stomach toward the spleen. A main duct, or channel, connects the pancreas to the duodenum.

ALERT

Anyone who takes insulin should have an emergency glucagon injection kit on hand. Glucagon is a hormone that prompts the liver to release glycogen and convert it into glucose. Glucagon is used to treat a severe hypoglycemic episode, or low blood sugar, in someone who has lost consciousness.

Pancreatic Tissues

In the pancreas, specialized cells known as *exocrine tissue* secrete digestive enzymes into a network of ducts that join the main pancreatic duct and end up in the duodenum. These enzymes are key in processing carbohydrates, proteins, and other nutrients.

The endocrine tissues of the pancreas contain cell clusters known as *islets of Langerhans*, named after Dr. Paul Langerhans, who first described them in medical literature. Islets (pronounced *EYE-lets*) are constructed of three cell types:

- **Alpha cells** manufacture and release glucagon (pronounced *glue-co-gone*), a hormone that raises blood glucose levels.
- **Beta cells** monitor blood sugar levels and produce glucose-lowering insulin in response.
- **Delta cells** produce the hormone somatostatin, which researchers believe is responsible for directing the action of both the beta and alpha cells.

Another Key Player: The Liver

Located toward the front of the abdomen near the stomach, the liver is the center of glucose storage. This important organ converts glucose—the fuel that the cells of the human body require for energy—into a substance called *glycogen*. Glycogen is warehoused in muscle and in the liver itself, where it can later be converted back to glucose for energy with the help of the hormone epinephrine (secreted by the adrenal glands) and glucagon from the pancreas. Together, the liver and pancreas preserve a delicate balance of blood glucose and insulin, which are produced in sufficient amounts to both fuel cells and maintain glycogen storage.

Insulin and Blood Sugar

While the liver is one source of glucose, most of the glucose the body uses is manufactured from food, primarily carbohydrates. Cells then metabolize, or convert, blood glucose for energy. And insulin is the hormone that makes it all happen.

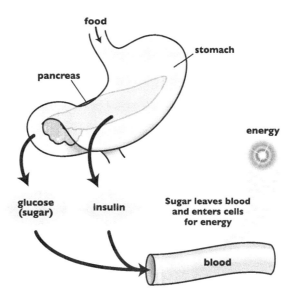

How it works: the pancreas, glucose, and insulin. Normally, insulin enters the bloodstream to regulate the levels of glucose.

To visualize the role of insulin in the body and in diabetes, think of a flattened basketball. The ball needs air (or glucose) to supply the necessary energy to bounce. To fill a basketball, you insert an inflating needle into the ball valve to open it, and then pump air through the needle into the ball. Likewise, when a cell needs energy, insulin binds to an insulin receptor, or cell gateway, to "open" the cell and let glucose in for processing. You can blow pounds and pounds of compressed air at the ball valve, but without a needle to open it, the air will not enter. The same applies to your cells. Without insulin to bind to the receptors and open the cell for glucose, the glucose cannot enter. Instead, it builds up to damaging and toxic levels in the bloodstream.

What Goes Wrong in Diabetes

In people with type 2 diabetes, the inflating needle (the insulin) is the wrong size or shape for the valve (the insulin receptor), or the valve itself is too small or missing. This phenomenon, where there's plenty of insulin but the body isn't using it properly, is known as *insulin resistance*.

As the beta cells try to produce more and more insulin in an effort to compensate for the body's growing inability to process glucose, another problem occurs. The pancreatic beta cells start to "burn out" and die, and *insulin insufficiency* (also known as insulin deficiency) is the result. The actual mechanics of how this occurs, and how early it happens in type 2, is not completely understood. But researchers have hypothesized that, at diagnosis, people with type 2 diabetes may have lost as much as 90 percent of their beta cell function.

FACT

Type 1 diabetes is different from type 2 diabetes. In type 1, the inflating needle is missing (no insulin production), or there are only one or two needles to fill an entire court full of basketballs (insufficient insulin production). This happens when the islets (specifically the insulin-producing beta cells) of the pancreas are destroyed.

Insulin resistance also occurs in gestational diabetes mellitus (GDM), a type of diabetes that first starts in pregnancy. Gestational diabetes usually resolves itself after childbirth, although women who develop GDM have a higher risk for another GDM diagnosis in future pregnancies. They also have an increased risk for developing type 2 diabetes later in life.

The Danger of High Blood Sugar

The human body needs glucose to function, but too much glucose circulating in the bloodstream has the potential to be toxic to all the tissues and organs of the body, including the insulin-producing beta cells of the pancreas. This is known as *glucotoxicity*. When insulin isn't available, blood sugar levels rise higher and higher in the bloodstream. A person may experience fatigue, excessive thirst, and increased urination. These are the classic symptoms many people develop before receiving a diabetes diagnosis.

A severe rise in blood sugar can result in diabetic ketoacidosis (DKA) or hyperglycemic hyperosmolar nonketotic coma (HHNC)—both are life-threatening medical emergencies. Timely diagnosis and treatment are important in preventing diabetes complications. Long-term, elevated blood sugars can damage virtually all the systems of the body. Blood vessel damage can result in cardiovascular disease, neuropathy (nerve damage), retinopathy (retinal eye disease), nephropathy (kidney disease), and more.

Managing Diabetes: A Balancing Act

While chronically high blood sugar levels cause diabetic complications over time, blood sugars that dip too low are also a problem. Hypoglycemia, or a low blood sugar level, is dangerous because, if left untreated, it can cause unconsciousness or even death. The most common triggers for a "hypo" include the following:

- An imbalance of food and insulin, such as when too much insulin is administered for the amount of carbohydrates eaten
- Certain type 2 oral medications
- Exercise without sufficient carbohydrate (carb) intake in individuals taking insulin and certain oral medications
- Excess alcohol intake without food in individuals taking insulin and certain oral medications

Some people who take insulin also experience overnight dips in blood glucose levels.

ESSENTIAL

A normal, nonfasting blood glucose reading is between 60 and 140 mg/dl (or 3.3 to 7.8 mmol/l). By contrast, the following glucose readings may indicate diabetes: a casual (i.e., any time of day) plasma glucose reading of 200 mg/dl (11.1 mmol/l) or higher, accompanied by high blood sugar symptoms; an A1C of 6.5 percent or higher; a fasting plasma glucose reading of 126 mg/dl (7.0 mmol/l) or higher; or an oral glucose tolerance test with a two-hour postload value of 200 mg/dl (11.1 mmol/l) or higher.

Controlling Blood Sugar

The ultimate goal of management of any type of diabetes is to bring blood sugar to a level that is as close to normal as possible, as consistently as possible. The American Diabetes Association (ADA) suggests adults with diabetes try to achieve blood sugar levels of 70 to 130 mg/dl (milligrams per deciliter) or 3.9 to 7.2 mmol/l (millimoles per liter) before meals, and less than 180 mg/dl (10.0 mmol/l) one to two hours after eating (i.e., postprandial). The American Association of Clinical Endocrinologists (AACE) suggests slightly different goals of less than 110 mg/dl (6.1 mmol/l) for a fasting blood glucose level and less than 140 mg/dl (7.7 mmol/l) two hours after meals.

It's important to remember, however, that each patient has unique blood sugar treatment targets. Those who are particularly susceptible to episodes of hypoglycemia may have slightly higher goals than those who aren't, while women who are trying to bring their glucose levels down as part of a pre-conception plan for pregnancy may have a lower target (i.e., need tighter control). Everyone is different, and your doctor will need to work with you to figure out what goals are right for you.

Treatment Tools

How do you bring blood sugars down to a controlled range? Although each person will have his or her own unique treatment plan, the main tools are diet, exercise, and medication. Proper nutrition and exercise should be a cornerstone of both disease management and healthy living. People with type 2 diabetes can sometimes control their disease with a combination of dietary regulation and exercise, but often they require pills, insulin, or other injectable medications.

What's in a Name?

Diabetes is the Greek word for "siphon" (since people with the disease tend to urinate copiously). *Mellitus* is Latin for "honey" or "sweet," a name added when physicians discovered that the urine from people with diabetes is sweet with glucose.

As researchers began to understand diabetes better, different subtypes of the disease were created. In 1980, the World Health Organization (WHO) recognized these types as insulin-dependent diabetes mellitus (or IDDM; type 1) and noninsulin-dependent diabetes mellitus (NIDDM; type 2). This classification scheme proved to be problematic because it defined diabetes not by the cause of the disease, but by its treatment—specifically whether or not a patient required insulin injections. This was often a cause for confusion because so-called noninsulin-dependent (type 2) patients often need insulin therapy to achieve good control.

FACT

Long before the advent of diagnostic urine testing in the nineteenth century, one of the earliest ways physicians learned to make a diagnosis of diabetes was to taste a patient's urine. Sugar in the urine produces a sweet taste.

▼ TYPES AND SUBTYPES OF DIABETES

Classification	Includes These Clinical Subtypes
Type 1	Type 1A, LADA (latent autoimmune diabetes in adults), Idiopathic type 1B
Type 2	N/A
Gestational	N/A
Other types, caused by the following:	Genetic defects and syndromes; Diseases of or injury to the pancreas; other endocrine disorders; drugs or toxins

Also confusing was the old-school system of calling type 1 diabetes "juvenile diabetes" and type 2 diabetes "adult-onset diabetes." While most cases of type 1 diabetes are diagnosed when patients are in childhood and adolescence, adults of any age, from twenty-somethings to the elderly, can develop the disease. And as obesity rates have soared in the United States in recent years, type 2 diabetes has begun to appear in younger adults, adolescents, and children. In short, there are no age limits to either type of diabetes. In the late 1990s, both the American Diabetes Association and the World Health Organization recommended using the names "type 1 diabetes" and "type 2 diabetes" as the clinical standard to distinguish these very complex and similar, yet very different diseases. However, you may come across a few doctors, and many laypeople, who still use the old names.

CHAPTER 2

Type 2 Diabetes

Type 2 diabetes, the most common type of diabetes, is also one of the most prevalent chronic diseases around. Worldwide, over 329 million people suffer from type 2 diabetes; and the International Diabetes Federation projects that by the year 2030 this population will reach nearly a half billion people. While excess body weight is a major risk factor for type 2 diabetes, ethnic background, family history, and certain components of an individual's health history also play important roles.

Insulin Resistance and Type 2

Type 2 diabetes is a metabolic disorder in which blood sugar rises because insulin does not effectively balance and metabolize the blood sugar into cell energy. The similarities in physiology between the two forms of diabetes end there, however.

ALERT

One of the reasons for the boom in type 2 diabetes in the United States and throughout the world is the widening of waistbands and the trend toward a more sedentary lifestyle. In the United States, the shift has been dramatic: In 2010, more than one-third of adults and nearly 17 percent of children between the ages of two and nineteen were classified as obese.

Type 2 diabetes is caused by the body's inability to use insulin properly. Two conditions that contribute to type 2 diabetes are *insulin resistance* and *insulin deficiency*. The first, insulin resistance, occurs in people who can produce insulin, usually in sufficient amounts at first. But when it's time for the insulin to bind to the insulin receptor—the gateway to cells in muscle, fat, and liver tissue—and initiate chemical signaling that allows the glucose in to be metabolized into cellular energy, something goes wrong. The insulin does not bind and so insulin resistance results. In other words, it's like trying to fit a square peg (insulin) into a round hole (insulin receptor). As a result, glucose doesn't enter the cells, and instead it builds up in the bloodstream, which results in high blood sugar levels.

The second condition that contributes to type 2 diabetes, insulin deficiency, occurs when the beta cells of the pancreas also have difficulty producing enough insulin to process the rising blood sugar levels. Eventually, the pancreas does not have sufficient amounts to overcome the deficit.

Research indicates that people with prediabetes already have an up to 70 to 80 percent decrease in beta cell function before they even cross the threshold into type 2 diabetes. After diagnosis, inflammatory processes in the body and the toxic effects of long-term high blood sugar levels on the beta cells on the pancreas (glucotoxicity) make insulin deficiency worse. Drug therapy is eventually required to preserve or recover beta cell function.

Prediabetes

Type 2 diabetes does not strike without warning. Prediabetes, also known as impaired glucose tolerance (IGT) or impaired fasting glucose (IFG), precedes the diabetes condition by months, years, and sometimes even decades. An estimated 79 million Americans have prediabetes; worldwide, that number is an estimated 280 million individuals. And many of these people are unaware of their condition.

FACT

Prediabetes affects 35 percent of adults twenty years old and older. And half of adults age sixty-five and older have prediabetes.

As the name suggests, prediabetes is defined by blood sugar levels that are higher than normal, but not high enough to indicate diabetes. The actual clinical criterion for a diagnosis of prediabetes is a fasting plasma glucose level of 100 mg/dl (5.6 mmol/l) to 125 mg/dl (6.9 mmol/l) or a two-hour plasma glucose level of 140 mg/dl (7.8 mmol/l) to 199 mg/dl (11.0 mmol/l), or a HbA1c value of 5.7–6.4 percent. Prediabetes signifies that without some healthy lifestyle changes, an individual is most certainly on the path to full-fledged type 2 diabetes. Prediabetes is a danger in itself: It increases the likelihood of stroke and heart disease by 50 percent.

Are You at Risk?

There are a number of known risk factors for both prediabetes and type 2 diabetes. If you have one or more of the following risk factors, you should be tested for prediabetes:

- Being overweight or obese (BMI of 25 or higher)
- Family history of diabetes (especially a first degree relative)
- Low HDL, or "good," cholesterol (less than 35 mg/dl, or 0.9 mmol/l) and high triglycerides (higher than 250 mg/dl)
- High blood pressure (consistent reading of 140/90 mmHg or higher)
- History of cardiovascular disease
- History of gestational diabetes

- History of polycystic ovary syndrome (PCOS)
- Giving birth to a baby weighing more than 9 pounds
- A previous hemoglobin A1C test result of 5.7 percent or higher
- Belonging to one of the following minority groups: African Americans, Native Americans, Hispanic Americans/Latinos, and Asian Americans/Pacific Islanders

Progression to Type 2 Diabetes

The pancreas of a person with type 2 diabetes generates insulin, but the body is unable to process it in sufficient amounts to control blood sugar levels. This inability is due to a problem with how the body's cells—specifically the insulin receptors that attract and process the hormone—recognize and use insulin. As blood sugar levels rise, the pancreas pumps out more and more insulin to try and compensate. This pumped insulin may bring down blood sugar levels to a degree, but it also results in high levels of circulating insulin, a condition known as *hyperinsulinemia*. At a certain threshold, the weakened pancreas cannot produce enough insulin; and over time beta cell mass is lost. As beta cells die, the insulin deficiency develops. At this point, type 2 diabetes results.

Risk Factors

The biggest indicator for your risk of type 2 diabetes is the diagnosed presence of prediabetes. But because the vast majority of people with prediabetes remain undiagnosed, assessing the presence of the other common risk factors for type 2 diabetes is important.

ESSENTIAL

While everyone with type 2 diabetes has some degree of insulin resistance, not everyone with insulin resistance has type 2 diabetes. Metabolic syndrome is a constellation of features—insulin resistance, low HDL and high LDL and triglycerides, excess abdominal fat, and high blood pressure—that put you at risk for heart disease.

Age and Ethnicity

According to the CDC, well over half of all cases of type 2 diabetes occur in people over age fifty, and nearly 11 million Americans age sixty-five and older suffer from the disease. Individuals over age forty-five should be tested for diabetes, and retested every three years thereafter if the initial test is normal. If you have additional risk factors for type 2 diabetes, you may require more frequent screening—talk to your doctor about your particular screening needs.

Certain ethnic groups and minorities have an increased risk of developing type 2 diabetes, including the following:

- African Americans
- Asian Americans
- Hispanics
- Pacific Islanders
- Native Americans

Family History

Heredity plays a large part in the development of type 2 diabetes. If you have a first-degree relative with type 2 diabetes, your chances of developing the disease double. There is a concordance rate of up to 90 percent among identical twins with type 2, meaning that in up to 90 percent of cases where one twin has the disease, the other one develops it as well.

The good news for those with diabetes in their family is that environmental factors such as your activity levels, health habits, and diet do play a large role in whether or not you will develop type 2 diabetes. Large-scale studies such as the Diabetes Prevention Program (DPP) have proven that prevention is often possible through eating well, exercise, and other moderate lifestyle changes. Adults in the DPP cut their risk of getting type 2 by over half by adding thirty minutes of exercise five days a week and changing their diet, showing that healthy living can overcome genetics in some cases.

Hypertension and Cholesterol Levels

Hypertension, or blood pressure of 140/90 mmHg or higher, is a known risk factor for the development of type 2 diabetes, and is also a frequent comorbid (i.e., coexisting) condition of the disease. A large-scale study of over 12,000 patients published in the *New England Journal of Medicine* found that people with diagnosed hypertension were 2.5 times more likely to develop type 2 diabetes than those individuals with normal blood pressure levels. In addition, that study and others have shown a correlation between beta-blockers, a medication used to treat high blood pressure, and an increased risk of type 2 diabetes.

Triglyceride levels over 250 mg/dl and/or levels of HDL (or "good cholesterol") under 35 mg/dl put you at an increased risk for type 2 diabetes. HDL acts as a lubricant for the circulatory system, moving the other lipids (triglycerides and LDL cholesterol) through the blood vessels and into the liver for metabolism. HDL helps to prevent the buildup of fatty plaque that can otherwise clog the arteries, resulting in atherosclerosis and, consequently, high blood pressure. Elevated triglycerides are also associated with an increased risk of heart disease.

Gestational Diabetes and Perinatal Risk Factors

Women who had gestational diabetes mellitus (GDM) during their pregnancy are at an increased risk of developing type 2 diabetes. Five to ten percent of women with GDM will have type 2 diabetes after labor and delivery. And women with a history of GDM have a 40 to 60 percent chance of developing type 2 diabetes within five to ten years postpartum, with a 70 percent risk thereafter. Giving birth to a baby weighing over nine pounds is also considered a risk factor for later development of type 2 diabetes. Several studies have linked high birth weights (over 4,000 grams, or 8.8 pounds) to type 2 diabetes.

ALERT

Women who have a history of gestational diabetes should be vigilant about regular testing for diabetes (once every three years if glucose levels are normal postpartum, annually if they are not).

A number of studies have also associated a low birth weight (under 2,500 grams, or 5.5 pounds) with an increased risk for type 2 diabetes later in life, possibly due to poor fetal nutrition.

Risks Associated with Weight and BMI

Obesity rates have been on a steady rise over the past few decades. The U.S. Centers for Disease Control (CDC) estimates that over 36 percent of U.S. adults are obese. In addition, a growing number of children and adolescents are living with weight issues. According to the 2009–2010 National Health and Nutrition Examination Survey (NHANES), over 18 percent of adolescents over age twelve, 18 percent of six- to eleven-year-olds, and 12 percent of children between the ages of two and five are considered overweight.

For children and adults alike, being overweight or obese is a primary risk factor for developing prediabetes and type 2 diabetes. The U.S. Department of Health and Human Services (HHS) reports that over 80 percent of people with type 2 diabetes are clinically overweight.

Why Is Weight a Risk Factor?

Too much fat makes it difficult for the body to use its own insulin to process blood glucose and bring it down to normal circulating levels. The specifics are as follows:

- **Overweight people have fewer available insulin receptors.** When compared to muscle cells, fat cells have fewer insulin receptors where the insulin binds with the cell and "unlocks" it to process glucose into energy.
- **More fat requires more insulin.** The pancreas starts producing larger and larger quantities of insulin in order to "feed" body mass, and consequently insulin resistance turns into a Catch-22.
- **Excess blood sugar must be stored as fat, and excess fat promotes further insulin resistance.** Fat cells release free fatty acids (FFAs). During lipolysis (the breakdown of fat within cells), free fatty acids are released into the bloodstream, interfering with glucose metabolism. Abdominal fat appears to release higher levels of FFA.

Leptin, a hormone in fat cells that helps to metabolize fatty acids, has provided an important clue to the relationship between obesity and type 2 diabetes. Discovered by Rockefeller University researchers in 1995, leptin (after the Greek *leptos*, meaning "thin") plays a part in sending a satiety—or "all full"—signal to the brain to stop eating when body fat increases, and an "empty" signal when body fat is insufficient. It appears that a type of leptin resistance may lead to a situation where fatty acids are deposited instead of metabolized, leading to eventual insulin resistance. Leptin may also play a role in signaling the liver to release stored glucose.

FACT

Women of reproductive age who have developed polycystic ovary syndrome (PCOS) are at an increased risk for type 2 diabetes. PCOS is a hormonal disorder characterized by enlarged ovaries that contain fluid-filled cysts. Insulin resistance and impaired glucose tolerance are features of PCOS.

Your BMI

Obesity and body fat are measured by body mass index (BMI)—a number that expresses weight in relationship to height and is a reliable indicator of overall body fat. People with a BMI of 25 to 29.9 are considered overweight; those with a BMI of 30 or over are obese.

You should aim for a BMI of 18.5 to 24.9, which is considered normal.

BMI is calculated differently for children and for young adults ages two to twenty. A charting system called BMI-for-age compares each child's weight in relation to other children of the same age and gender on a growth chart in terms of percentiles. For example, a girl in the thirteenth percentile would weigh the same or more than 13 percent of girls the same age. A healthy BMI for children is from the fifth to less than the eighty-fifth percentile. Growth charts used for assessing pediatric BMI-for-age are based on National Health and Nutrition Examination Survey (NHANES) data and generated by the U.S. Centers for Disease Control and Prevention (CDC).

A BMI-for-age that is at the ninety-fifth percentile or higher is considered obese, while the eighty-fifth to less than the ninety-fifth percentile is overweight.

BMI	19	20	21	22	23	24	25	26	27	28	29	30	31	32	33	34	35	36	37	38	39
Height (inches)	Body weight (pounds)																				
58	91	96	100	105	110	115	119	124	129	134	138	143	148	153	158	162	167	172	177	181	186
59	94	99	104	109	114	119	124	128	133	138	143	148	153	158	163	168	173	178	183	188	193
60	97	102	107	112	118	123	128	133	138	143	148	153	158	163	168	174	179	184	189	194	199
61	100	106	111	116	122	127	132	137	143	148	153	158	164	169	174	180	185	190	195	201	206
62	104	109	115	120	126	131	136	142	147	153	158	164	169	175	180	186	191	196	202	207	213
63	107	113	118	124	130	135	141	146	152	158	163	169	175	180	186	191	197	203	208	214	220
64	110	116	122	128	134	140	145	151	157	163	169	174	180	186	192	197	204	209	215	221	227
65	114	120	126	132	138	144	150	156	162	168	174	180	186	192	198	204	210	216	222	228	234
66	118	124	130	136	142	148	155	161	167	173	179	186	192	198	204	210	216	223	229	235	241
67	121	127	134	140	146	153	159	166	172	178	185	191	198	204	211	217	223	230	236	242	249
68	125	131	138	144	151	158	164	171	177	184	190	197	203	210	216	223	230	236	243	249	256
69	128	135	142	149	155	162	169	176	182	189	196	203	209	216	223	230	236	243	250	257	263
70	132	139	146	153	160	167	174	181	188	195	202	209	216	222	229	236	243	250	257	264	271
71	136	143	150	157	165	172	179	186	193	200	208	215	222	229	236	243	250	257	265	272	279
72	140	147	154	162	169	177	184	191	199	206	213	221	228	235	242	250	258	265	272	279	287
73	144	151	159	166	174	182	189	197	204	212	219	227	235	242	250	257	265	272	280	288	295
74	148	155	163	171	179	186	194	202	210	218	225	233	241	249	256	264	272	280	287	295	303
75	152	160	168	176	184	192	200	208	216	224	232	240	248	256	264	272	279	287	295	303	311
76	156	164	172	180	189	197	205	213	221	230	238	246	254	263	271	279	287	295	304	312	320

Normal   Overweight   Obese

Body mass index (BMI) table

Body Shape

Having an apple-shaped body, with excess pounds packed in the midsection rather than the hips, is another hallmark of insulin resistance. In fact, the National Institutes of Health recommends that waist circumference be used as a screening tool for evaluating the risk of heart disease and type 2 diabetes.

▼ **CLASSIFICATION OF OVERWEIGHT AND OBESITY BY BMI, WAIST CIRCUMFERENCE, AND ASSOCIATED RISK OF TYPE 2 DIABETES, HYPERTENSION, AND CARDIOVASCULAR DISEASE**

Disease Risk Relative to Normal Weight and Waist Circumference			
BMI (kg/m2)		≤102 cm. (≤40 in.) for men; ≤88 cm. (≤35 in.) for women	>102 cm. (>40 in.) for men; >88 cm. (>35 in.) for women
Underweight	<18.5	no increased risk	no increased risk
Normal	18.5–24.9	no increased risk	no increased risk
Overweight	25.0–29.9	increased	high
Obesity	30.0–34.9	high	very high
	35.0–39.9	very high	very high
Extreme Obesity	≥40	extremely high	extremely high

From the National Institutes of Health; National Heart, Lung, and Blood Institute

Another type 2 risk sometimes related to weight is an inactive lifestyle. Exercise, even at a moderate level, reduces blood glucose levels. People who lead sedentary lifestyles, exercising fewer than three times a week, are more likely to develop type 2 diabetes than those who are more active.

Signs and Symptoms

It's important to note that not all people with type 2 diabetes will have symptoms, particularly in the early stages of the disease. In fact, over a third of all Americans with type 2 diabetes are unaware that they have it. Often the first symptoms they notice, such as tingling or burning in the hands and feet (neuropathy) or slow-healing wounds, are actually complications caused by long-term uncontrolled blood sugar.

Symptoms of type 2 diabetes may include one or more of the following:

- Thirst and frequent urination
- Tingling or burning pain in the feet, legs, hands, or other parts of the body
- Fatigue, or a feeling of being run-down and tired
- Blurred vision
- Extreme hunger

- Unexplained weight loss
- Frequent or recurring infections (e.g., urinary tract infections, yeast infections)
- Slow healing cuts and bruises

Even though the signs of type 2 diabetes tend to develop gradually, it's important to see your doctor right away if you experience any of these symptoms. Left unchecked, rising blood sugars will cause steady damage to your body. And any kind of infection—urinary tract, ear, viral, etc.—can cause blood sugar to rise further and has the potential to trigger a life-threatening diabetic emergency such as diabetic ketoacidosis (DKA) or hyperglycemic hyperosmolar nonketotic syndrome (HHNS).

Diabetic Ketoacidosis (DKA)

When blood glucose levels in an individual are extremely high (above 250 mg/dl or 13.9 mmol/l), signs of DKA may start to appear. Ketoacidosis is a life-threatening condition and requires immediate medical attention. Symptoms and signs of DKA include the following:

- Lethargy
- Nausea and vomiting
- Abdominal pain
- Fruity breath odor
- Rapid breathing
- Dehydration
- Ketones in the blood and urine
- Loss of consciousness

DKA must be treated in the hospital with intravenous insulin therapy. If you develop DKA at the diagnosis of type 2, you may be taken off insulin once your health and blood sugar has stabilized and put on metformin or other oral diabetes drugs.

Hyperglycemic Hyperosmolar Nonketotic Syndrome (HHNS)

When an individual's blood glucose levels exceed 600 mg/dl (33.3 mmol/l), a condition known as hyperglycemic hyperosmolar nonketotic syndrome (HHNS) may occur. In HHNS, the body becomes severely dehydrated. Older adults tend to develop HHNS more readily, although the condition can occur at any age. HHNS is a life-threatening condition and requires immediate medical attention.

Indications of the syndrome include the following signs and symptoms:

- Excessive thirst
- Fever
- Dizziness or feeling faint
- Disorientation and/or sleepiness
- Visual disturbances and/or hallucinations
- Hemiplegia (paralysis or weakness on one side of the body)
- In extreme cases, coma

Diagnosing Type 2 Diabetes

A blood test is used to diagnose type 2 diabetes. A normal, nonfasting blood glucose reading is between 60 and 140 mg/dl (3.3–7.8 mmol/l). The following readings may indicate type 2 diabetes: an A1C test of 6.5 percent or higher; a casual plasma glucose reading of 200 mg/dl (11.1 mmol/l) or higher (accompanied by symptoms of hyperglycemia); a fasting plasma glucose reading of 126 mg/dl (7.0 mmol/l) or higher; or an oral glucose tolerance test with a two-hour postload value of 200 mg/dl (11.1 mmol/l) or higher.

FACT

Maturity-onset diabetes of the young (MODY) is a form of diabetes caused by a specific genetic defect of beta cell function. Although MODY is often treated like type 2 diabetes (with diet, exercise, and occasionally, oral medications), it is a distinctly different class of diabetes.

Long-term uncontrolled blood sugar levels can cause major damage to virtually every system in the body, head to toes. If you are experiencing any of the symptoms of diabetes, it's crucial that you visit a health care professional as soon as possible for evaluation. If you are diagnosed as having diabetes, maintaining tight control of your blood sugar levels is the best way to avoid serious complications.

Not Just for Adults Anymore

Type 2 diabetes, once considered an adults-only disease, is appearing in children and teens in epidemic proportions. The National Diabetes Education Program estimates that children comprise nearly half of the newly diagnosed cases of type 2 diabetes. Certain ethnic minority children are disproportionately affected by type 2; Native Americans are at highest risk, followed by Asian-Pacific Islander, African American, and Hispanic children.

This alarming surge in childhood type 2 diabetes has been fueled by a fast food diet and a sedentary lifestyle. It is a lifestyle that is centered around passive entertainment media, such as television and online gaming, and supersized, high-calorie convenience foods that have no real dietary value. As a result, according to the U.S. CDC nearly 17 percent of children and adolescents age nineteen and younger are obese, which puts them at high risk for impaired glucose tolerance and insulin resistance.

Kids at Risk

The same factors that place adults at great risk for type 2 diabetes apply to children as well. Obesity is by far the primary threat in this age group.

ESSENTIAL

Acanthosis nigricans (darkening of the skin) is a sign of insulin resistance that appears in up to 90 percent of children and adolescents who develop type 2 diabetes. These dark, velvety patches typically appear in areas where skin folds gather (e.g., neck, armpits, groin) and are more common in people with darker skin pigmentation.

Having a family history of type 2 diabetes among first- and second-degree relatives and being of African American, Native American, Asian, or Hispanic descent also increase the likelihood that these overweight children will develop the disease.

The majority of childhood type 2 cases are diagnosed at puberty or in adolescence. Puberty itself is the cause of a certain degree of insulin resistance in adolescents, which is thought to be triggered by a natural rise in growth hormone during this time. In children who are already disposed toward the disease, insulin resistance remains even after growth hormone returns to normal levels.

Treating Kids for an Adult Disease

Diagnoses of type 2 in children are sometimes difficult to make, especially in children who are not overtly obese. Many physicians still consider type 2 diabetes an adults-only disease. Often because of the age of the patient, type 1 is initially suspected and the child begins insulin treatment. However, long-term use of insulin after blood sugars have stabilized can contribute to further weight gain for the patient, which can worsen the problem.

QUESTION

My daughter is overweight, but we have no history of diabetes in our family. Should I really be concerned about her weight?
Yes. Weight problems in childhood can lead to the development of a host of medical problems, such as atherosclerosis, hypertension, respiratory infections, sleep apnea, and type 2 diabetes. Talk to her pediatrician about a weight-loss strategy. And remember, diet and exercise should become a family affair to ensure the greatest chance of success for your daughter.

Children diagnosed with type 2 diabetes can usually be treated through a combination of diet and exercise. Oral medications may be helpful, but clinical data is limited on their long-term effects in children. As of mid-2012, metformin was the only oral agent approved for use in pediatric populations (over age ten) by the U.S. Food and Drug Administration (FDA). However, other oral agents are sometimes prescribed for off-label use in children.

Off-label use is when a medication is prescribed for an indication, or purpose, other than what it has been approved for by the FDA.

A Word on LADA

Statistically speaking, most diabetes cases diagnosed in adults turn out to be type 2 diabetes. However, in some cases diabetes that strikes in adulthood is actually a form of type 1, or "juvenile" diabetes.

LADA, or latent autoimmune diabetes in adults, occurs in up to 10 percent of all cases of diagnosed type 2 diabetes of adults over age thirty. LADA and type 2 diabetes are very different conditions that require different treatment approaches. But because both conditions are diagnosed in adulthood and present with the same symptoms and gradual onset, and because type 2 diabetes is so widespread in the U.S. population, there is a high degree of misdiagnosis between LADA and type 2 diabetes patients.

Over time, misdiagnosis can lead to sudden life-threatening high blood sugars; so it's important for adults who do not fit the classic profile of type 2 diabetes and who cannot get their blood sugars under control to be tested for LADA.

LADA can be distinguished from type 2 diabetes through blood tests for autoantibodies such as GAD (glutamic acid decarboxylase) and levels of c-peptide, a protein that is a byproduct of insulin production. The GAD antibody is an enzyme that is produced when inflammatory processes in the body start destroying the pancreatic beta cells. Low levels of c-peptide also indicate problems with insulin production.

FACT

LADA is actually a subtype of type 1 diabetes that has a very gradual onset. This immune-mediated form of diabetes is also referred to as late-onset autoimmune diabetes of adulthood, slow-onset type 1, or type 1.5 diabetes. People with LADA rarely need insulin injections at first. And because of this slow onset, they are often misdiagnosed with type 2 diabetes.

If you are over age thirty and can answer yes to two or more of the following questions, you could have LADA:

- You have no family history of type 2 diabetes
- You are at or near your ideal weight for your height (neither overweight nor obese)
- You have another autoimmune condition or a family history of another autoimmune condition (e.g., thyroid disease, celiac)
- You are not able to keep your blood sugar under control despite sufficient effort and treatment adjustments to your diet, exercise regime, and/or oral medicines

If you suspect that you could have LADA, talk to your doctor about appropriate screening tests.

CHAPTER 3

You Have Diabetes . . . Now What?

A diagnosis of diabetes is a scary thing, but a knowledgeable and communicative health care team can make the ride a little less bumpy. Your doctor is only one part of the equation—because diabetes is a systemic disease that can affect every part of your body, you'll also be seeing a team of specialists who will help you prevent and treat complications. If you choose them thoughtfully and play an active and educated role in your care, then you will be in charge of your diabetes rather than the other way around.

Making the Diagnosis

Diabetes is diagnosed through a lab test that measures the level of glucose in your blood. Because a rise in blood sugar levels might be attributable to some other factor, such as illness or stress, a second blood test is usually performed the following day to establish the diagnosis.

FACT

The normal range for the fasting plasma glucose test (FPG) is considered to be less than 100 mg/dl (5.6 mmol/l). Those with FPG results between 100 mg/dl (5.6 mmol/l) and 125 mg/dl (6.9 mmol/l) are said to have prediabetes.

There are four different types of diagnostic blood tests available for diabetes: the hemoglobin A1C, the fasting plasma glucose test, the oral glucose tolerance test, and the random plasma glucose test. This last test, the random plasma glucose, should only be used if obvious symptoms of hyperglycemia (i.e., high blood sugar) are present. In most cases, no matter what the test, confirmation of the diagnosis with a second test is recommended to rule out any lab error.

The Hemoglobin A1C Test (A1C)

In recent years, the A1C blood test has become a common diagnostic tool for diabetes and prediabetes. This test does not require you to fast, and it provides a quick and easy way for health care providers to get a clear picture of your average blood sugar levels over the past three months.

The A1C test may be done in the doctor's office or in a lab. An A1C of 6.5 or higher is diagnostic of diabetes. If no symptoms of diabetes are present, the diagnosis should be confirmed by an A1C test.

Your doctor will continue to use this test after diagnosis to see how you are doing with blood sugar control. Information about regular A1C screening to meet and stay at target is addressed elsewhere in this book.

Fasting Plasma Glucose Test (FPG)

The FPG is a carbohydrate metabolism test that measures plasma (blood) glucose levels after a fast of at least eight hours. Fasting stimulates the release of the hormone glucagon, which in turn raises plasma glucose levels by triggering the breakdown of glycogen (stored glucose) in the liver. In people without diabetes, the body will produce and process insulin to counteract this rise in glucose levels. With diabetes, this does not happen, and the tested glucose levels will remain high.

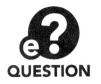

QUESTION

Can the OGTT be used to diagnose prediabetes?
Yes, both the FPG and the oral glucose tolerance test (OGTT) can be used to diagnose prediabetes. Individuals with two-hour plasma glucose OGTT results between 140 mg/dl (7.8 mmol/l) and 199 mg/dl (11.0 mmol/l) are said to have impaired glucose tolerance (IGT).

The fasting plasma glucose test should be administered in the morning because, aside from the fact that it is easiest to fast during sleeping hours, blood glucose tests given in the afternoon tend to provide lower readings and could miss some cases of prediabetes and diabetes. According to ADA clinical practice guidelines, a fasting reading of 126 mg/dl (7.0 mmol/l) or higher indicates diabetes, and a second follow-up oral glucose tolerance test on a subsequent day should be performed to confirm the diagnosis if symptoms of diabetes are not present. The OGTT is considered a more sensitive (albeit more time-consuming and expensive) test than the FPG.

Oral Glucose Tolerance Test (OGTT)

The OGTT is a test that measures blood glucose at one-hour intervals over a two-hour period. The patient is given a 75-gram drink of glucose solution, which should cause blood sugar levels to rise in the first hour, and then fall back to normal within the second hour as the body produces more insulin to normalize glucose levels.

Blood drawn two hours after drinking the glucose solution (also called two-hour postload blood draw) that has glucose levels of less than 140 mg/

dl (7.8 mmol/l) is considered normal. Two-hour postload levels of 140 mg/dl (7.8 mmol/l) or higher but less than 200 mg/dl (11.1 mmol/l) are an indication of impaired glucose tolerance (prediabetes). Blood sugar levels of 200 mg/dl (11.1 mmol/l) or higher two-hour postload point to type 2 diabetes and should be confirmed by a second OGTT or FPG test on a different day if symptoms of diabetes are not present.

ALERT

Home A1C test kits are available at your local pharmacy and other retail outlets. However, not all of these tests meet the ADA-mandated assay lab standards for A1C and diabetes diagnosis. You should never use these home tests to try and self-diagnosis diabetes. If you suspect that you or someone you care for has diabetes, take them to a health care professional for appropriate testing and evaluation.

Random or Casual Plasma Glucose Test

The random plasma glucose test, also called a casual plasma glucose test, can be given at any time of the day, regardless of whether the patient has eaten or not. This test is recommended for diagnosis only if symptoms of high blood sugar, such as excessive thirst or urination, are present. Random plasma glucose levels of 200 mg/dl (11.1 mmol/l) or higher, along with symptoms of hyperglycemia, are considered diagnostic of diabetes. A second test on another day is recommended to confirm the diagnosis if numbers are high but symptoms are not present.

After a diagnosis is made, further lab tests may be ordered to determine the progression of your disease and the possibility of coexisting conditions that are common in diabetes.

▼ **ADA GUIDELINES FOR DIAGNOSING DIABETES**

Test	Normal Levels	Prediabetes	Diabetes*
Fasting plasma glucose	<100 mg/dl (5.6 mmol/l)	100 (5.6 mmol/l) to 125 mg/dl (6.9 mmol/l)	≥126 mg/dl (7.0 mmol/l)
Hemoglobin A1C	< 5.7 percent	5.7–6.4 percent	≥6.5 percent

Test	Normal Levels	Prediabetes	Diabetes*
Oral glucose tolerance test**	<140 mg/dl (7.8 mmol/l)	140 (7.8 mmol/l) to 199 mg/dl (11.0 mmol/l)	≥200 mg/dl (11.1 mmol/l)
Casual plasma glucose			≥200 mg/dl (11.1 mmol/l) in the presence of symptoms

*Diagnosis should be confirmed with a test on a subsequent day

**Two-hour postload readings

C-Peptide Test

If your doctor is unsure whether you have type 1 or type 2 diabetes, a c-peptide test may be ordered. C-peptide is one component of the molecule proinsulin (the other component is insulin itself). The levels of c-peptide in your bloodstream can help establish how much insulin your pancreas is still able to produce.

C-peptide can also diagnose hyperinsulinemia (high levels of circulating insulin) in type 2 diabetes. The normal range for c-peptide levels varies, as several different laboratory methods of performing the test exist. Ask your physician for assistance in interpreting your specific results.

Conditions such as pregnancy or renal failure can affect c-peptide levels, as can certain medications and alcohol intake. Also, the test should not be performed immediately following a glucose tolerance test (GTT), as a GTT can elevate c-peptide levels.

Other Tests

If you are a new patient, your physician will take a detailed medical history at your initial visit. You should also undertake a thorough, head-to-toes physical examination to check for the presence of possible complications of diabetes. This examination should include an evaluation of your cardiac (heart) function, blood pressure, and a neurological examination of your reflexes and ability to recognize certain types of stimulation.

A monofilament test, which involves touching the bottom of your foot with a piece of fiber that resembles a thick strand of fishing line, is an easy and inexpensive way to establish if you have lost sensation in your feet due to nerve damage—a condition called peripheral neuropathy.

Your feet will also be examined carefully for infection, ulceration, and circulatory problems. A weak pedal pulse (pulse taken on the foot) may be an early sign of peripheral vascular disease, or PVD. PVD is a condition where the blood vessels in the extremities (usually the feet) become narrowed or blocked and, as a result, blood flow is reduced to the surrounding tissues.

Other tests that may be performed at or shortly following your initial diagnosis include the following:

- A urine test for microalbumin, a protein that can indicate problems with kidney function
- A fasting blood lipid profile, to check cholesterol and triglyceride levels
- Electrocardiogram (ECG or EKG), to assess cardiac function

Additional tests and procedures may also be indicated, depending on your specific medical history.

Choosing a Doctor

Once you have a confirmed diagnosis, it's time for you to take a step back and make a decision about who will be your partner in managing your diabetes. If you have a doctor who communicates well, listens to your thoughts and concerns, and seems up to speed on current developments in diabetes care, you may decide to stay with her. However, if your doctor-patient relationship is more on the dysfunctional side, it may be time for you to shop around for someone new. Here are a few questions to consider:

- **Does your physician provide cutting-edge care?** Is she current on the latest clinical studies, new products, and treatment guidelines?
- **Is your doctor willing to listen and learn?** Does she let you voice questions and concerns and give you a chance to ask follow-up questions?
- **Is she reasonably available?** How does she handle daytime and after-hours phone calls from patients? Does she return calls in a timely manner?

- **Does she treat the person, not just the disease?** Does her treatment philosophy reflect a good understanding of the social and emotional impact of diabetes? Does she ask questions about your lifestyle to make sure your treatment plan is working?
- **What's her bedside manner like?** Is she abrupt with her staff? Does she brush off patient questions? Do you want a person who just isn't nice to be your treatment partner for the lifelong commitment of diabetes management?
- **Does she tell it like it is?** Having a doctor who explains tests and treatment decisions is essential. She should be able to communicate with you frankly and in terms you can understand.

Remember, your doctor is only one member of your health care team, albeit an important one. She should communicate well with other members of the team as well as with you—sharing information and getting consultation on treatment decisions when appropriate (for instance, working with a neonatologist or ob-gyn to discuss pregnancy issues).

Do You Need a Specialist?

You may need to get a new doctor who specializes in diabetes if your health care picture is complex, or if you or your physician don't feel comfortable with his level of expertise in diabetes care. An endocrinologist is a doctor who specializes in gland and hormone disorders. He may work with a variety of endocrine disorders or focus specifically on diabetes. *Diabetologist* is another name for a physician—endocrinologist, internist, or otherwise—who specializes in diabetes care. Children with diabetes may also benefit from the expertise of a pediatric endocrinologist (or pediatrician with a special expertise in the management of diabetes).

ESSENTIAL

Many people with diabetes continue to see a general practitioner after diagnosis. As long as your doctor has experience treating diabetes, stays up-to-date on the latest in diabetes care, is a good partner in your treatment, and communicates well, it really doesn't matter what initials follow your doctor's name.

Some people choose to continue to see their internist or general practitioner for regular health care checkups and nondiabetes-related ailments, and visit an endocrinologist for diabetes care. If you go this route, encourage your health care providers to communicate and share information openly. Remember, you are the head of your health care team.

Communication Is Key

So exactly what defines good communication? It's talking with each other rather than at each other—listening instead of just hearing and explaining rather than commanding. If you ask your doctor why he has ordered a certain test, he should be able to explain his decisions to you in nontechnical language. And if your doctor has questions about your self-care, you should be forthright and honest so he can provide you with the best care possible. The following suggestions may help you improve communication between you and your doctor:

- Think about the symptom(s), questions, and treatment issues you want to discuss in advance. Bring notes if necessary.
- Bring your medications (in their original bottles) with you for doctor visits. This should include herbs and supplements—your doctor should know what you're taking because some supplements may interact with other medications or may be inappropriate for diabetes patients.
- Treat your doctor as you would like to be treated—respectfully and candidly.
- Bring someone else along to join you after the examination to hear what the doctor recommends.
- Take your pills as prescribed; if you are not taking your pills, let your doctor know.
- Don't be a "no-show" for appointments, and let the scheduler know exactly what the purpose of the visit is so that she can book your appointment for an appropriate length of time.

Remember, if you don't understand what your doctor is telling you, ask questions. Even after you leave your appointment, don't hesitate to pick up the phone and ask questions. It's important that you fully comprehend how you are supposed to be treating your diabetes.

Your Health Care Team

Diabetes is a systemic disease that has the potential to affect every part of your body, so preventive care by a team of trained experts is an absolute essential. In addition to your primary care doctor, you may be seeing a number of specialists.

Your primary care physician may be able to provide initial screening for diabetes-related complications, but she may also refer you to another doctor who has specialized training in a given area of concern. Ophthalmologists, mental health providers, nephrologists, and podiatrists are just a few of the other care providers who can help you stay healthy and avoid complications.

Ophthalmologists and Retinologists

The blood vessel damage associated with diabetes puts you at risk for diabetic retinopathy and other vision problems. Ideally, you should see a medical doctor (MD) who is trained in eye diseases—an ophthalmologist—to treat any existing eye disease and to screen for possible problems. You may also choose to visit a retinologist—an ophthalmologist with specialized training in retinal diseases.

An optometrist (an eye care professional who is not a physician) may also provide screening services for diabetic retinopathy. The ADA recommends an annual dilated-eye exam for all people with type 2 diabetes. The initial exam should be conducted shortly after diagnosis. Your doctor may recommend less frequent exams after several normal eye exams, or more frequent checks should you develop signs of retinopathy.

Mental Health Professionals

The psychological toll of diabetes can also be a tremendous burden on you, both emotionally and physically. People living with diabetes are twice as likely to experience depression. Left untreated, depression can inhibit your ability to effectively manage your diabetes. Therapists, psychiatrists, psychologists, and/or trained counselors can help you cope with the stresses of diabetes. Support groups are a great resource for helping you come to grips with diabetes, and also enable you to learn from the experiences of others.

Nephrologists

Because diabetes is the number one cause of chronic kidney disease, you may see a nephrologist—a physician specializing in renal care. For patients whose kidney disease progresses to ESRD (end-stage renal disease), a nephrologist will also be in charge of prescribing dialysis treatments.

Podiatrists

Proper foot care and regular foot exams are extremely important in diabetes care. For this reason, a podiatrist, or foot doctor, may also be a key member of your diabetes health care team. Podiatrists can detect and treat neuropathy (nerve damage) of the feet and foot ulcers. These specialists can also help educate you on preventive foot care.

FACT

Laws governing patient access to medical records vary by state. Some health care providers may only release records to physicians rather than directly to you. Other providers may charge a fee to cover the costs of copying and retrieving patient files. Check with your state department of health to obtain the policies in your area.

Other Team Players

Other specialists who may be on your health care team include the following:

- **Gastroenterologist:** A physician who specializes in diseases and disorders of the digestive tract
- **Gynecologist:** A doctor who specializes in women's reproductive medicine

- **Obstetrician:** A physician who monitors pregnancy and birth
- **Urologist:** An MD with special training in treating the urinary tract
- **Neurologist:** A specialist of the central nervous system and brain who treats central nervous system (CNS) disorders such as neuropathy (nerve damage)
- **Dermatologist:** A doctor who treats skin diseases and disorders, and may have special training in wound care
- **Physical therapist:** A trained health care professional who assists in strength and mobility recovery through exercise and other techniques

Coordinating Care

Good communication is essential for coordinating the activities of a team of specialists treating your diabetes and related complications. In an ideal world, all of your doctors would quickly follow up with your primary physician and promptly consult with other specialists when your medical problems extend outside of their particular area of expertise. In reality, you may face missing lab reports, contradictory treatment recommendations, and other obstacles.

Short of hiring a personal secretary to keep track of what can be a complex medical schedule and a rapidly expanding file of charts, there are a few things you can do to ensure that all your providers are working effectively as a team. If your primary care provider referred you to a specialist, call at least forty-eight hours before your appointment to make sure the new physician has all the clinical information she needs from your regular doctor. And when you go to your appointment, ask the specialist what her office procedure is for following up with your primary provider.

Here's what else you can do:

- Offer to deliver treatment reports from specialists to your primary care provider and vice versa.
- Ask for hard copies of lab results and diagnostic tests so you have a backup and don't waste a trip to the doctor's office if they don't get delivered.
- Keep a running list of all medications that your various physicians prescribe and bring the list to your doctors' appointments.

- Take notes of questions, concerns, and new issues raised at your appointments so you can share them with your primary care provider.

Remember, your health care providers work for you, but you are ultimately in charge of your own health care. Don't be shy about following up on your treatment, and don't let any doctor or medical staff make you feel guilty about doing so. If they do, it may be time to consider finding someone new.

Getting a Good Education

Since you spend most of your time away from the doctor's office, it's important to learn as much as you can at home about how you can manage your diabetes and prevent complications. In fact, diabetes is such a complex disease that it merits its own course of study. Self-care, a generalized term for looking after yourself and promoting wellness, is the main thrust of diabetes education. You must also learn essential skills, such as testing your blood sugar levels and injecting insulin.

ESSENTIAL

Diabetes education classes are usually geared toward people who are newly diagnosed with the disease, although there are some "refresher" courses for people who have lived with diabetes for some time or who want to learn ways to better control their blood sugar levels.

Going to School

Your doctor can refer you to classes in your area and, in fact, should offer you information on diabetes education at or shortly following your diagnosis. Classes are often held at local hospitals or freestanding clinics, and are typically covered by most health insurance plans (check with your insurer on your eligibility). In addition, your doctor may have diabetes educators who work at his practice.

Diabetes classes cover a wide range of issues, including how diabetes physically and emotionally affects your body, how to test blood sugars, the importance of exercise, knowing the signs of a blood sugar emergency, regulating medications and/or insulin, recognizing and preventing complications, and coping with lifestyle issues. Another primary teaching point is diet management.

Diabetes education classes are typically taught by a diabetes nurse educator or dietitian educator. Most likely, the instructor will be a certified diabetes educator (CDE). Educators with the CDE designation have completed specific training in diabetes patient education. Classes range from short workshops to intensive, multipart courses. There are also CDEs who work one-on-one with patients. Again, your doctor can provide a referral, or you can contact the American Association of Diabetes Educators (AADE) to locate a CDE in your area at *www.diabeteseducator.org*.

Food Savvy RDs

Dietary management is one of the cornerstones of diabetes care. A registered dietitian (RD) or a nutritionist who works with patients with diabetes is an essential member of your care team. An RD can teach you concepts like carbohydrate counting and can explain how certain foods affect blood sugar levels. These professionals can also help you achieve any weight loss goals.

Most important, your dietitian can also work with you one-on-one to design a meal plan that fits your particular lifestyle. For example, if you're a vegetarian, it will do you little good to get a menu that features fish and meat. Or if, for example, you have a job that keeps you out on the road a great deal of the time, you need someone who can help you make healthy choices outside of your kitchen. Consulting with an RD allows you to develop menus that are based in reality. If your diet is practical, then you're more likely to follow it and stick to it in the long term.

Taking Control

Is your head spinning yet? With all the information thrown at you, both in class and by well-meaning friends and relatives (who quite frequently spread misinformation rather than fact), feeling overwhelmed is completely normal. Take a deep breath and remember three things:

1. You aren't in this alone—your health care team is there to help.
2. You don't have to learn it all at once—control involves some trial and error.
3. Reinventing the wheel is not necessary—others have gone before you, and you'll get through the physical and emotional demands much easier if you join a support group and draw on their wisdom.

In diabetes-care lingo, *control* is maintaining blood sugar levels as close to normal (nondiabetic) levels as much of the time as possible. The ADA recommends that people with diabetes aim for blood sugar levels of 70 to 130 mg/dl (3.9 to 7.2 mmol/l) before meals and less than 180 mg/dl (10.0 mmol/l) after meals (that is, one to two hours after the start of a meal). The American Association of Clinical Endocrinologists (AACE) suggests slightly different goals of <110 mg/dl (6.1 mmol/l) before meals and <140 mg/dl (7.8 mmol/l) two hours after meals.

It is important to remember that these are general recommendations only, and you will work with your doctor to determine the blood sugar goals that are right for you and your particular health picture. And remember, while there are many guidelines and targets in diabetes care, nearly everything about the disease varies by individual. A food that sends one person's blood sugar off the charts may cause barely a ripple for another.

A Treatment Triad

People living with type 2 diabetes sometimes are able to use only diet and exercise to effectively keep their blood sugar levels under control. But often, a little help from oral medications, insulin, or other injectable drugs is also required. Needing medication to control your diabetes doesn't make you any less successful at managing your disease than someone who is able to do it through diet and exercise only. Together, diet, exercise, and medication are simply different tools designed to help you achieve the same goal— better blood sugar control.

Eat Right

It is essential that you know how food choices affect your blood sugar. More than 80 percent of people with type 2 diabetes are overweight or obese; and for these people, eating for both blood sugar control and weight loss is often a fundamental component of their self-care. Appropriate food choices and dietary considerations for diabetes, also called medical nutrition therapy (or MNT), are covered in detail elsewhere in this book.

Exercise

Exercise is fundamental to good health and well-being. It lowers blood sugar levels, improves heart health, and promotes weight loss in overweight people. However, people with diabetes must take precautions with their exercise routine to ensure that they don't experience a blood sugar low.

Medication

The latest ADA clinical practice guidelines recommend that, along with lifestyle changes, most people with type 2 diabetes start metformin, a diabetes pill, at the time of their diagnosis. The exception would be anyone with an allergy to the drug or other conditions not compatible with the drug (like kidney failure). For those with critically high blood sugar levels at diagnosis, insulin therapy is suggested instead.

However, given time, in some cases people are able to successfully manage their type 2 diabetes through diet and exercise, particularly with weight loss. It's important to keep in mind, however, that type 2 diabetes is often a progressive disease. Insulin resistance and beta cell death increase with age, meaning that many people with type 2 will eventually need the additional assistance of oral or injectable medications at some point in their lives. This course of treatment isn't a sign of failure, but of the natural progression of the disease.

Standards of Care

In today's health care environment, doctor appointments, tests, and treatments are frequently dictated by the bottom line of your insurance company. However, many insurance providers recognize the value of increasing their investment in preventive care to avoid bigger bills down the road. In other words, diabetes treatment may cost a lot, but the price tag on treatment of diabetic complications, such as chronic kidney disease, blindness, and heart attack, is even higher.

FACT

Both the American Diabetes Association (ADA) and the American Association of Clinical Endocrinologists (AACE) have issued clinical practice recommendations for diabetes care. U.S. providers look to these recommendations as professional guidelines for the diagnosis and treatment of diabetes.

You will probably see your doctor more frequently immediately following your diagnosis, as you work to normalize your blood sugar levels. Once you've found a treatment routine that works for you, the time between visits may be extended to quarterly or possibly twice a year. If you change your medication or insulin routine, your team will want to monitor you more closely for a period of time.

Setting Your Goals

When you are managing any chronic health condition, especially one that touches so many facets of your lifestyle, like diabetes, it's important to have goals to work toward. Goals not only help you measure progress, they can be incredibly empowering and motivational when they are set and tracked correctly.

However, the wrong kind of goal setting can have the opposite effect. Goals that are unrealistic, too vague, or don't hold you to any timeline for completion may actually work against you.

It may sound counter-intuitive, but it may be helpful to initially set your sights low. If you aim for the stars relative to your starting point, you may become easily discouraged if you don't hit that big goal as quickly as you feel you should.

S.M.A.R.T. Goals

In the long run, the most effective goals are S.M.A.R.T. goals. What's a S.M.A.R.T. goal?

1. **<u>Specific.</u>** Don't be vague or general. Saying "I will eat healthier" leaves a lot of room for interpretation. But saying "I will add one more serving of

a low-carb veggie to my meals each day for a week" is a concrete objective you can achieve.

2. **Measurable.** Make sure your goals can be measured against something. Whether it's testing three more times a week or exercising twenty additional minutes a day, putting a number against your goal helps you ensure you're making progress.

3. **Action oriented.** It may go without saying, but your goal should require you to do something to achieve it. Goals aren't wishes; they are something to work toward by taking tangible steps.

4. **Realistic.** Don't set goals that you know, deep down, you don't stand any chance of achieving. Do not set goals you are simply not capable of making or goals that require too much drastic change at once. A realistic goal is something you are fairly certain you can achieve in the short term.

5. **Timely.** Set a time limit for your goal. Starting with a short time period can be a good motivator for sticking to your goal. As you experience success meeting it, you can always extend the time frame longer.

▼ GOALS: WHAT WORKS AND WHAT DOESN'T

Not so S.M.A.R.T.	What's Missing	The S.M.A.R.T. Version
I will test my blood sugar more.	Not measurable or timely.	I will test my blood sugar one more time each day for two weeks.
I will start exercising.	Not specific, measurable, or timely.	I will walk for 20 minutes at least three days a week for a month.
I will lose 50 pounds this month.	Not action oriented or realistic.	I will lose 3–5 pounds in a month by following the eating and exercise plan I developed with my registered dietitian.
I will take better care of myself.	Not specific, measurable, or timely.	By the end of this month, I will make an appointment for my annual dilated eye exam, and I will ask for a reminder call for next year's appointment.
I will have fewer blood sugar swings this month.	Not action oriented.	I will log my sugars, food, meds, and exercise for two weeks and bring it to my doctor to look for patterns that could be causing my blood sugar swings.

Start by picking one goal for yourself. If you're having problems figuring out what the best goal is for you to start with, you can work with your doctor or diabetes educator to narrow down the options.

When You Meet Your Goals

What's the best thing to do once you've met a S.M.A.R.T. goal? Get S.M.A.R.T.E.R., of course. That means *evaluating* and *resetting* your goals. Look at the progress you've made with the original goal. How well did you do in achieving it? Are you satisfied with the results? Are there any changes you could make to do better the next time around in terms of being specific, measurable, action oriented, realistic, and timely?

If you feel the goal you've worked toward and met has become a healthy new lifestyle habit, then it's time to move on to a brand new goal (with S.M.A.R.T. goal setting in mind, of course). But if your achieved goal isn't quite habit yet, or if the time frame for your goal has elapsed without quite meeting the measurement you set for yourself, you might consider resetting to the same goal—with any modifications you figured out while evaluating your success (e.g., set a different time frame, determine a change in measure).

Remember that you can evaluate and reset goals at any point in time if you feel like you aren't making adequate progress. Goals should always be a work in progress. And you should always be working toward a goal, even if you've reached your target A1C. Doing so will help you stay motivated toward maintaining good diabetes health and prevent you from becoming complacent.

CHAPTER 4

Food and Blood Sugar

The food you eat has a big influence on your blood sugar levels and therefore on your diabetes control and risk of related complications. In fact, what you eat is so important that the ADA refers to dietary management of diabetes as medical nutrition therapy (MNT). To be successful at MNT, you need to learn about carbohydrates and good diabetes food choices.

All about Carbohydrates

Carbohydrates are your body's primary source of glucose, and glucose is your cellular fuel. The body begins to convert carbohydrates almost entirely into glucose shortly after carb-containing foods are eaten. Insulin helps to "unlock" the cells to move the glucose from the bloodstream into the cells for energy. If you have insufficient insulin production or your body is resistant to insulin, consuming too many carbohydrates can cause blood sugar to rise.

All foods that contain starches and/or sugars—including fruits, vegetables, milk, yogurt, breads, grains, beans, and pasta—contain carbs. Virtually the only whole foods that are carbohydrate-free are protein-rich meats, poultry, finfish (when prepared without additional ingredients such as breading and marinades), and fats such as cooking oils and shortening. To avoid all carb-containing foods is both impossible and unadvisable—your body needs the important micronutrients and phytochemicals contained in these foods. But you do need to learn the basics of assessing the quantity and quality of carbohydrates in your food, how your body reacts to them, and how to make smart carb choices based on this information.

Carb Science

Carbohydrates are categorized by their chemical structure. A monosaccharide, or simple sugar, is composed of a single saccharide (sugar) chain. Glucose, fructose (fruit sugar), and galactose are all simple sugars. Disaccharides are two simple sugars joined together, and include lactose (milk sugar), maltose (malt sugar), and sucrose (table sugar). Polysaccharides, or complex carbohydrates, are ten or more simple sugar chains joined. Glycogen, starches, and fiber are polysaccharides. (A fourth type of carbohydrate, oligosaccharides, is composed of three to ten sugar chains, but most of these are usually formed from the breakdown of polysaccharides.)

ESSENTIAL

The glycemic index (GI) of foods does not necessarily correspond to a specific carbohydrate "type"—some complex carbs may have a higher GI than simple carbs. For people with diabetes, the GI can be an effective tool for avoiding blood sugar spikes.

All carbohydrates must be hydrolyzed, or broken down, into monosaccharides before the body can process them. Amylase, a type of enzyme found in the saliva and secreted by the pancreas, helps to break down carbs into glucose during their journey through the small intestine. Once hydrolysis occurs, the resulting glucose is absorbed into the bloodstream. Any excess glucose is converted to glycogen and stored in the liver, along with fructose and galactose.

The Glycemic Index

Does it matter what kind of carbs you consume? At one time, nutritionists believed that people with diabetes should avoid simple sugars (monosaccharides and disaccharides) and eat foods that contain complex carbohydrates instead. This recommendation was founded on the mistaken belief that simple sugars would raise glucose levels faster and more dramatically across the board. But it's now known that gram for gram, the complex carbohydrates found in breads, cereals, potatoes, vegetables, and other foods raise blood sugar approximately the same amount as do simple sugars like honey, fructose, or table sugar. However, there may be a difference in how rapidly certain foods raise blood sugar levels. The glycemic index (or GI) is a measure of how quickly the carbs in certain foods are transformed into blood glucose. Foods with a low GI (e.g., beans, multigrain bread) raise glucose levels at a slower and steadier rate than a high-GI food (e.g., rice, potatoes).

ALERT

People with gastroparesis, or nerve damage of the stomach, have delayed stomach-emptying issues that can delay or prolong the normal blood glucose rise from the carbohydrates they eat. If you have gastroparesis or other gastrointestinal/digestive issues, make sure your dietitian is aware of them when working out a meal plan with you.

Carbs and Blood Glucose Control

Carbohydrates and the glucose they generate are an energy source—the dietary fuel of the human body. Insulin produced by the pancreas enables our cells to burn this carb-generated glucose. This is why determining the amount of carbohydrates in a meal is so important for blood sugar control.

People who take mealtime insulin have to inject enough insulin to accommodate, or "cover," all the carbohydrates they eat. Many people with diabetes must also adjust their diets in an effort to lose excess weight. Concepts like carbohydrate counting and dietary exchanges (covered in Chapter 5) enable people with diabetes to effectively manage their blood sugar levels.

It's important to understand that carbohydrates don't work in isolation. Other nutrient components of the food you eat also can affect your body's ability to absorb carbs. High-fat and high-protein foods can delay carb absorption. And although fiber is considered a carbohydrate, high-fiber foods also slow the absorption of glucose because they slow the passage of food through the digestive tract.

Why Fiber Is Important

Fiber, or roughage, is composed from plants' cell wall material. Whole grains, legumes (dried beans and peas), nuts, and vegetables are all good sources of dietary fiber. Fiber is considered a carbohydrate, but since the body cannot digest the majority of fiber, it does not effectively contribute to a rise in blood sugar levels. In fact, dietary fiber is an important nutritional tool in normalizing blood sugar levels because it slows digestion and therefore the absorption of accompanying nutrients.

ALERT

Always consume plenty of water or caffeine-free beverages—at least 2 liters, or around eight glasses, daily—if you are eating a fiber-rich diet. The consumption of fiber without adequate fluid intake can lead to constipation. Increasing fiber intake slowly can also help to ease any bloating or other unwanted gastrointestinal distress.

How It Works

When viscous (water-soluble) fiber absorbs water in the gastrointestinal tract, it turns to a gel-like substance that helps to normalize blood glucose and insulin levels by slowing the passage of food through the intestines. The delay in nutrient absorption means a slower and more stable rise in blood glucose levels. Because soluble fiber absorbs the excess intestinal bile acids that help to form cholesterol, soluble fiber in turn helps lower blood cholesterol levels, which is another important consideration for people with diabetes who are at risk for cardiovascular disease. Viscous fiber also improves satiety, or the feeling of fullness you get when eating. That is, viscous fiber delays stomach emptying, and in those people with type 2 diabetes who are also overweight, satiety can be a useful tool for achieving weight loss.

Recommended Intake

A diet high in low-glycemic whole-grain cereal fiber has been found to have a beneficial effect in controlling postprandial (after-meal) blood glucose levels and for reducing serum cholesterol levels in people with type 2 diabetes. Some studies have shown a glucose- and lipid-lowering benefit with fiber intake of up to 50 grams daily. The ADA recommends a daily fiber intake of at least 14 grams per 1,000 calories. Talk to your doctor and dietitian about what level of fiber in your diet is right for you.

ESSENTIAL

In the United States, carbohydrate information on food labels includes total dietary fiber. When counting carbs for the nutritional management of diabetes, most dietitians recommend that you subtract the total grams of dietary fiber from the total carbohydrates in those foods that contain more than 5 g of fiber per serving.

Fiber intake has also been associated with a reduction in diabetes risk in a number of studies. One of these studies, the six-year Nurses' Health Study, involved more than 65,000 participants and found that women on a low-fiber diet that was heavy in processed, sugary foods were 2.5 times more likely to develop type 2 diabetes than those who ate at least 25 grams of fiber daily.

The Facts about Sugar

The no-sugar myth is probably one of the biggest misconceptions about diabetes. The reality is that it isn't sugar specifically that raises blood glucose levels—it's any food that contains carbohydrates, including honey, fruit, milk, bread, and vegetables, to name a few. So whether it's a spoonful of sugar, a bagel, or a banana, it will cause blood sugar levels to rise. However, some foods may cause a faster or more pronounced blood sugar spike (see the glycemic index section in Chapter 5).

So sugar isn't, in itself, completely off-limits in a diabetes meal plan. However, moderation in sugar intake is important. Some people with diabetes prefer to use sugar substitutes such as artificial sweeteners or sugar alcohols because they contain few or no carbohydrates or calories.

Sugar Alcohols

A sugar alcohol is, quite simply, a monosaccharide that has been chemically transformed into its alcohol form. A number of naturally occurring sugar alcohols (also called polyols) are available, including sorbitol, mannitol, xylitol, lactitol, maltitol, isomalt, erythritol, and hydrogenated starch hydrolysates. Because they are not completely absorbed in the gastrointestinal tract, they don't cause much of a rise in blood glucose levels, which is why people with diabetes may find them desirable. Polyols are frequently used as sweeteners and bulking agents in processed foods marketed as sugar-free.

ALERT

Because children have a lower tolerance for sugar alcohol sweeteners, check the labels of "sugar-free" foods carefully and be cautious with the amount of sugar alcohols your child consumes. If your child is sensitive to sugar alcohols, there are other artificial sweeteners available that don't cause gastrointestinal side effects.

Some people find that sugar alcohols have a laxative effect, causing diarrhea and/or gas. The U.S. Food and Drug Administration requires that foods containing significant amounts of sorbitol or mannitol (food products that, when consumed, may result in over 50 grams of sorbitol or 20 grams of mannitol) must be labeled with the statement: "Excess consumption may have a laxative effect."

When calculating carbohydrates in foods that contain sugar alcohols, you should subtract half of the sugar alcohol grams (located on the nutrition label) from the total carbohydrate count.

Artificial Sweeteners

As opposed to naturally derived sugar alcohols, artificial sweeteners include the following synthetically manufactured sugar substitutes:

- **Aspartame (NutraSweet or Equal):** This FDA-approved sweetener is 180 times sweeter than table sugar. Aspartame has been the subject of much controversy regarding its potential negative health effects. However, there is currently no clinical research to indicate that this sweetener is unsafe for most people (except for individuals with advanced liver disease, pregnant women, and those with a rare genetic condition known as phenylketonuria, or PKU).
- **Neotame:** This sweetener is derived from aspartic acid and phenylalanine (both are amino acids). Neotame is considered safe for use by people with diabetes, children, pregnant and lactating women, and individuals with PKU. It is primarily used in food manufacturing.
- **Saccharin (Sweet'N Low):** The oldest artificial sweetener, saccharin was discovered in 1879 and has been used as a sweetener in foods and beverages for over a century. Saccharin has been linked to bladder cancer in rats, but there is no hard data to establish that normal amounts of the sweetener are dangerous for humans. In 2000, based on a newer and more relevant body of human studies, the National Toxicology Program of the National Institutes of Health took saccharin off its ninth edition of the Report of Carcinogens list; and President Clinton signed legislation removing the carcinogenic warning label from saccharin-containing products. Saccharin is considered GRAS (generally recognized as safe) by the FDA and is about 300 times sweeter than table sugar.
- **Acesulfame potassium (Sunett):** Acesulfame potassium, also called acesulfame K, is FDA approved for use as a sweetener in processed foods and beverages. It is an estimated 200 times sweeter than table

sugar, and studies have confirmed its safe use for people with diabetes, pregnant and nursing women, children, and the general population.

- **Sucralose (Splenda):** Sucralose is unique in that it is derived (through a chemical process of chlorination) from table sugar. However, unlike table sugar, it has no carbohydrates, no calories, and it passes through the body almost entirely undigested. This sugar substitute, which is 600 times sweeter than table sugar, was cleared by the FDA for use as a food additive and a sweetener in the late 1990s. Because it is very stable and withstands temperature changes well, it can be used in cooking and baking. Extensive clinical studies have uncovered no safety risks for people with diabetes and the general population.

Some artificial sweeteners are available in special blends that combine the sweetener with sugar. These blends are marketed for use in baking and cooking and are designed to add texture and color to foods. When using a sweetener blend, be sure to check the nutrition facts label carefully for the total carbohydrate count per serving.

A Few Words on Stevia

The herb stevia is said to be 200 to 300 times sweeter than table sugar and is derived from the herb *Stevia rebaudiana*, a wild shrub that is grown in South America and the Pacific Rim. It has no carbohydrates and does not raise blood sugar levels. Often touted as the natural alternative to other chemically based sugar substitutes, the herb has had a rough road gaining regulatory acceptance in the United States.

The FDA initially banned the import of stevia in 1991, following a study that raised questions about its toxicity as a food additive. But subsequently, the FDA allowed it to be sold as a dietary supplement. In 2008, the FDA allowed food manufacturers to file for GRAS status for food products made with Rebaudioside A (or Reb A). Reb A is a highly purified extract of the stevia herb. This extract has a body of substantial, controlled research to back up its safety. The result is that tabletop sweeteners containing this stevia extract can now be sold as food products, not supplements, for the first time.

Other foods and beverages sweetened with Reb A can be found on your grocery store shelves. It is important to note that whole leaf stevia and other stevia extracts are still not FDA approved for use in food products in the

United States, and can only be found as supplements. If you're considering using a supplement form of stevia, talk with your doctor and dietitian before incorporating it into your food plan.

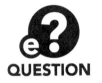

If a food is sugar-free, does that mean I can eat as much as I want? Don't be misled by a "sugar-free" label. Foods containing polyols and/or artificial sweeteners may still contain carbohydrates and calories that should be figured into your meal plan. Read the nutrition facts on the label to get the full story.

Caloric Intake

Ideal calorie intake is based on your activity level, gender, age, and other factors. Many people with type 2 diabetes also face weight-loss challenges; since reducing calorie intake is one component of an effective weight-reduction program, it is an important consideration in the dietary management of diabetes.

The following are estimated amounts of daily calorie intake based on gender, age, and activity levels from the U.S. Department of Agriculture's "2010 Dietary Guidelines for Americans." These general guidelines are for weight maintenance, not weight loss.

▼ **ESTIMATED DAILY CALORIE INTAKE**

Gender/ Activity Level*	Male/ Sedentary	Male/ Moderately Active	Male/ Active	Female**/ Sedentary	Female**/ Moderately Active	Female**/ Active
Age (years)						
2	1,000	1,000	1,000	1,000	1,000	1,000
3	1,200	1,400	1,400	1,000	1,200	1,400
4	1,200	1,400	1,600	1,200	1,400	1,400
5	1,200	1,400	1,600	1,200	1,400	1,600
6	1,400	1,600	1,800	1,200	1,400	1,600
7	1,400	1,600	1,800	1,200	1,600	1,800
8	1,400	1,600	2,000	1,400	1,600	1,800

Gender/ Activity Level*	Male/ Sedentary	Male/ Moderately Active	Male/ Active	Female**/ Sedentary	Female**/ Moderately Active	Female**/ Active
Age (years)						
9	1,600	1,800	2,000	1,400	1,600	1,800
10	1,600	1,800	2,200	1,400	1,800	2,000
11	1,800	2,000	2,200	1,600	1,800	2,000
12	1,800	2,200	2,400	1,600	2,000	2,200
13	2,000	2,200	2,600	1,600	2,000	2,200
14	2,000	2,400	2,800	1,800	2,000	2,400
15	2,200	2,600	3,000	1,800	2,000	2,400
16	2,400	2,800	3,200	1,800	2,000	2,400
17	2,400	2,800	3,200	1,800	2,000	2,400
18	2,400	2,800	3,200	1,800	2,000	2,400
19–20	2,600	2,800	3,000	2,000	2,200	2,400
21–25	2,400	2,800	3,000	2,000	2,200	2,400
26–30	2,400	2,600	3,000	1,800	2,000	2,400
31–35	2,400	2,600	3,000	1,800	2,000	2,200
36–40	2,400	2,600	2,800	1,800	2,000	2,200
41–45	2,200	2,600	2,800	1,800	2,000	2,200
46–50	2,200	2,400	2,800	1,800	2,000	2,200
51–55	2,200	2,400	2,600	1,600	1,800	2,200
56–60	2,200	2,400	2,600	1,600	1,800	2,200
61–65	2,000	2,400	2,600	1,600	1,800	2,000
66–70	2,000	2,200	2,600	1,600	1,800	2,000
71–75	2,000	2,200	2,600	1,600	1,800	2,000
76+	2,000	2,200	2,400	1,600	1,800	2,000

Based on Estimated Energy Requirements (EER) equations, using reference heights group. For children and adolescents, reference height and weight vary. For adults, the reference woman is 5 feet 4 inches tall and weighs 126 pounds. EER equations are from the Institute of Medicine. Dietary Reference Intakes for Energy, Carbohydrate, Fiber, Fat, Fatty Acids, Cholesterol, Protein, and Amino Acids. Washington (DC): The National Academies Press; 2002.

*Sedentary means a lifestyle that includes only the light physical activity associated with typical day-to-day life. Moderately active means a lifestyle that includes physical activity equivalent to walking about 1.5 to 3 miles per day at 3 to 4 miles per hour, in addition to the light physical activity associated with typical day-to-day life. Active means a lifestyle that includes physical activity equivalent to walking more than 3 miles per day at 3 to 4 miles per hour, in addition to the light physical activity associated with typical day-to-day life.

**Estimates for females do not include women who are pregnant or breastfeeding.

Source: Britten P, Marcoe K, Yamini S, Davis C. Development of food intake patterns for the MyPyramid Food Guidance System. J Nutr Educ Behav 2006;38(6 Suppl):S78-S92.

It's More Than Just the Calories

If you are overweight and have type 2 diabetes, keep in mind that even modest weight loss can decrease insulin resistance and improve control. But calorie reduction alone as a weight loss strategy rarely leads to long-term weight control. The ADA suggests a comprehensive approach of reduced calories (500 to 1,000 fewer calories than the USDA guidelines listed for weight maintenance), regular exercise, reduced fat intake (no more than 30 percent of daily calories from fat), and diabetes and weight management education. In their most recent Clinical Nutrition Recommendations, the ADA also recognized the utility of low-carbohydrate diets in weight loss.

The nutrient balance in the food your calories come from is also important. The ADA suggests that 15 to 20 percent of your caloric intake should be protein, while no more than 7 percent of total calories should come from saturated fat.

Fats and Cholesterol

Fat insulates the body and supplies energy when no carbohydrate sources are available. It also enables the body to absorb and process the fat-soluble vitamins A, D, E, and K. However, some types of fat and cholesterol may increase the risk of atherosclerosis and other cardiovascular complications from diabetes.

ALERT

Food with high fat and/or high protein levels can delay the absorption of carbohydrates, and consequently delay the postprandial (after-meal) rise of blood glucose. People who take insulin need to be especially aware of this phenomenon. Pizza is one food that is well known for causing this "delayed reaction" in people with diabetes.

All Fats Are Not Created Equal

Fats are confusing to many people when they first start learning about the dietary management of diabetes. The off-target message that "all fat is bad" has become entrenched in popular dietary culture; and fat-free food production is now a multimillion-dollar industry. While some fats are bad for you in excess, others can actually help improve your cholesterol profile. Here are the basics on dietary fats:

- **Saturated fat:** Solid fats that are found in meat and dairy products and vegetable oils. Too much saturated fat in the diet may be associated with high LDL (bad) cholesterol levels. However, research is conflicting as to whether or not dietary saturated fat actually increases your risk of heart disease, and recent studies dispute this claim.
- **Unsaturated fat:** Either polyunsaturated (e.g., safflower oil) or mono-unsaturated (e.g., olive oil); found in fish and seafood, among other sources. These types of fats (polyunsaturated in particular) have been shown effective in reducing total and LDL (bad) cholesterol levels.
- **Trans fats/hydrogenated fats:** Transunsaturated fatty acids, or unsaturated liquid fats that have been processed into a more saturated and solid form by adding hydrogen. These fats are often found in processed baked goods and commercial fried foods, and may be called partially hydrogenated or hydrogenated fats. Trans fatty acids can raise LDL (bad) cholesterol and lower HDL (good) cholesterol, and their use should be limited or avoided altogether.
- **Essential fatty acids:** Fish and fish oils and certain seeds and nuts and their oils (e.g., flaxseed, canola, soybean, and walnut) are all good sources of omega-3 fatty acids, which have heart-protective benefits and lower both triglyceride levels and blood pressure. Linolenic, alpha-linolenic, eicosapentaenoic, and docosahexaenoic acids are all essential fatty acids.
- **Dietary cholesterol:** Cholesterol is present in food that comes from animals, including poultry, fish, eggs, meats, and dairy products.

Less than 7 percent of daily calories should come from saturated fats, and trans-fat intake should be limited as much as possible. Cholesterol intake should be less than 200 milligrams per day. The ADA also recommends two or more servings of fish weekly for the cardioprotective benefits of omega-3 fatty acids.

Fake Fats

Fat substitutes and replacers are food additives derived from protein, carbohydrates, or chemically modified fat. They are designed to replace the texture, moisture-retention, and bulk of fat in food while providing a lower amount of calories. The main pitfall of reduced-fat and fat-free foods is that some people interpret the label as meaning calorie-free, and so they overindulge. And in some cases, fat substitutes (e.g., dextrose, cellulose) are filled with added carbohydrates, which can result in higher blood sugar for people with diabetes.

However, when prudently used, reduced-fat products can be a useful component of a weight-loss plan. Further studies are needed to determine the long-term impact of fat substitutes on overall calorie intake and nutrient absorption. Some fat substitutes, such as olestra (Olean), may inhibit the absorption of fat-soluble vitamins A, D, E, and K. The FDA has mandated that products made with olestra be fortified with these vitamins to overcome the deficit.

Protein and Diabetes

Proteins are chains of amino acids responsible for cell growth and maintenance and are found in virtually every part of the body. Protein in foods from animal sources (meat, poultry, fish, and dairy) is called *complete protein* because it contains essential amino acids necessary for building and maintaining cells. Protein in plant-based foods such as grains, beans, fruit, and vegetables is called *incomplete protein* because it contains only partial groups of these amino acids. However, different incomplete plant-based proteins can be combined to form complete proteins in the diet. If you are a vegetarian or vegan and have diabetes, a dietitian with experience in vegetarian menu planning can advise you on appropriate protein consumption choices.

People with diabetes should have 15 to 20 percent of total calories from protein, as is recommended for the general population. People with impaired kidney function, or nephropathy, may need to avoid a high protein diet because damaged kidneys cannot filter protein efficiently from the bloodstream. If you have kidney problems, talk to your doctor and dietitian about an appropriate level of protein for your diet.

Sensible Sodium Intake

In moderate amounts, dietary sodium or sodium chloride (salt) is not harmful. In fact, this mineral helps to maintain a healthy electrolyte balance and works in tandem with potassium to regulate blood acid/base balance, heart function, nerve impulses, and muscle contractions.

However, people with high blood pressure need to be cautious about having too much sodium in their daily diet. The Dietary Approaches to Stop Hypertension (or DASH diet) study found that limiting dietary sodium is associated with a substantial reduction in blood pressure in adults with hypertension. For most people with diabetes and hypertension, the ADA recommends a daily sodium intake of 2,300 milligrams, equivalent to a teaspoon of sodium chloride, or table salt. The average American, however, consumes more than twice that much. Watch out for added sodium in condiments and packaged and canned foods.

ESSENTIAL

Be salt-smart and check food labels. Be on the lookout for monosodium glutamate (MSG), sodium nitrite (nitrate), sodium caseinate, sodium alginate, sodium sulfite, sodium hydroxinate, sodium propionate, sodium saccharin, sodium bicarbonate (baking soda), and sodium benzoate. Even some multivitamins contain sodium.

Some people with diabetes and hypertension may benefit from an even bigger cut in dietary salt intake. A study published in the *New England Journal of Medicine* examined sodium intake in the Dietary Approaches to Stop Hypertension (DASH) diet and found that reducing sodium intake to 1,560 milligrams and 960 milligrams daily reduces blood pressure significantly when it is part of a comprehensive DASH diet—a dietary approach that is low in saturated fat and cholesterol and rich in fiber, protein, calcium, magnesium, and potassium. If you're having problems stepping away from the salt shaker, try kicking up the flavor with other herbs and spices that don't contain sodium. Experiment with new tastes and increase the percentage of unprocessed whole foods in your diet to keep yourself on track.

CHAPTER 5

Eating Right in Action

If you're looking for a "diabetic diet" full of bland, boring foods and completely devoid of any desserts, indulgences, or the other little taste treats that make life worth living, you are out of luck. The so-called diabetic diet is largely a myth; people with diabetes can and do enjoy a wide variety of foods, the same foods everyone else can eat. The key is moderation, a focus on healthier carb choices, and a keener awareness of how foods affect your blood sugars and body.

Menu Planning

A meeting with a registered dietitian (RD) is an absolute must for anyone with diabetes. A good RD will explain the mysteries of exchanges and carbohydrate counting to you and will work with you to create a meal plan that works with your lifestyle. If you don't have an RD already, talk to your doctor about a referral, or visit the Academy of Nutrition and Dietetics Association's online referral database at *www.eatright.org*.

As a member of your diabetes care team, your dietitian should be in close contact with your care provider. Make sure your RD is on top of any adjustments made to your insulin or medication, which go hand in hand with what you're eating. It helps to bring a spouse or companion for another set of ears when you go to the dietitian's office, particularly your first time there.

Whether you're using carbohydrate counting or dietary exchanges, your RD will try to spread out your carbohydrate intake more or less evenly throughout the day to promote blood glucose balance. Again, your dietitian will work with you to come up with an appropriate amount of exchanges of carb grams, fat intake, and protein. He may also suggest other dietary guidelines based on your health history (e.g., low sodium if you have hypertension).

QUESTION

How can I eat right when my wife brings junk food into the house for the kids?
Diabetes is a family disease. Ask your wife to join you for a diabetes education class and/or a meeting with your dietitian and discuss ways of promoting a healthier lifestyle for the entire family. Your children will also benefit from the same type of healthy meal plan you're following for your diabetes.

The ADA recommends that people with diabetes eat no less than 130 grams of carbs daily. However, many people with diabetes find that an even lower intake of carbohydrates offers them better control of their blood glucose levels. If you'd like to try a lower-carb meal plan, talk with your RD and your doctor about an approach that's right for you.

Finding Your Way with the Food Groups

You've been taught about the four basic food groups since childhood, and may be wondering how they fit into this diabetes equation. Here's the run down:

- **Fruits and Vegetables.** Filled with nutrients and good for you, fruits and veggies are definitely part of a healthy "diabetes diet." Dark leafy green veggies that are high in fiber are best, while starchy vegetables like potatoes should be eaten in moderation. Good low-carb choices include broccoli, green beans, spinach, kale, green peppers, asparagus, okra, cauliflower, and lettuce.

  Fruits contain natural sugars (fructose) that raise blood sugar levels, so choose ones that are high in fiber to moderate that effect. Watermelon, strawberries, grapefruit, blackberries, blueberries, honeydew melon, and avocado (yes, it's a fruit) are all choices that should be kind to your blood sugar levels. Like veggies, no fruits are off-limits, but those that are higher in carbs, like bananas, figs, mangoes, and grapes, should be eaten in small portions. And remember that all dried fruits (e.g., raisins, prunes, dates, dried apricots) are extremely high in sugar.

- **Breads and Cereals.** This is a tricky category. It's important to get some whole grains in your diet to promote good diabetes and heart health. Yet breads and cereals tend to be very high in carbohydrates and therefore not a great choice for keeping blood sugars steady. Checking the label is important. There should be at least 5 g of fiber, if not more, in a serving. Look at the nutrition facts panel for total carbohydrates as well, and comparison shop for a bread that has more fiber and fewer carbs.

  Avoid cereal products that contain sweeteners like high fructose corn syrup and even sugar, molasses, and honey. It's better for your blood sugar if you add your own sweetener, or a low-carb fruit, to an unsweetened cereal.

- **Dairy.** Both the ADA and the USDA recommend low-fat versus full-fat dairy products. Traditionally this recommendation has been based on the presumed link between saturated fat and heart disease. However, recent research, including a 2010 meta-analysis of twenty-one studies and nearly 350,000 subjects, has found that dietary saturated fat was not associated with an increased risk of coronary heart or vascular disease.

Whether or not saturated fat is the dietary culprit it has long believed to have been is a subject of hot debate in the nutrition world, and it will probably continue to be for some time. If your doctor, diabetes educator, or dietitian does recommend low-fat dairy to you, just keep in mind that low-fat food products often have added carbohydrates in the form of sugars or thickeners to improve their taste. As always, check the label for total carbohydrates and adjust your serving sizes accordingly.

- **Meat, Poultry, and Fish (Protein).** When prepared without sauces or breading, meat, poultry, and fish are all carbohydrate free. Choosing lean cuts of meat will help you avoid some of the added fat and calories. The ADA recommends two or more servings of fish a week for the heart-healthy omega-3 fatty acids it provides.

Dear Diary . . .

Even if you follow your meal plan to the letter, you're still going to find that certain foods will give you a bigger spike in blood sugar levels than expected. You may also find that other foods you expected to pump up your readings barely bump the meter. That's the individual nature of diabetes. For this reason, a food diary is an invaluable tool in figuring out just how different foods affect your blood glucose levels.

ALERT

As you learn how variations in food choices, timing of meals, and exercise affect your blood glucose levels, you and your dietitian and doctor can work together to fine-tune your carb-counting program. It is a learning process, so don't be disappointed if it doesn't fall into place immediately.

Record the type, amount, and timing of foods eaten, along with what effect they had on your blood sugar levels (a reading before eating and a reading two hours after). Many people choose to record the information in a blood sugar logbook. At first it may feel a little obsessive-compulsive to chronicle every bite, but you'll find it's worth it when the time comes to figure out a mysterious high or an unexpected low. It's also a great cure for mindless eating—you won't thoughtlessly polish off what the kids left on their dinner plate or munch samples in the supermarket if you've trained yourself to write it down.

Carbohydrate Counting

Most diabetes educators and registered dietitians teach carbohydrate counting as the primary method of maintaining dietary control of diabetes. Carb counting involves calculating the grams of carbohydrates eaten in a given meal. In theory, regulating carb intake means controlling your blood glucose levels.

How many carbohydrates you eat in a given day depends on your unique caloric, medical, and lifestyle needs. An active teenager will have a greater carbohydrate requirement than an inactive adult. Again, the first step in establishing a carb-counting plan is to sit down with a registered dietitian and discuss your medical history, lifestyle, eating habits, and medication routines, and then come up with a plan for how many carbohydrates you should be eating and when they should be consumed.

Choices Versus Grams

There are a couple of different variations on the carb-counting theme. One method is basic carb gram counting, which is to simply calculate the actual grams of carbohydrates you consume and ensure they don't exceed a pre-established limit. Another popular method is carb choice.

Since a dietary exchange of starch or fruit carbohydrates is equivalent to 15 grams of carbohydrates, many dietitians use the "15 grams per serving" value as a rule of thumb when teaching carb counting, especially to those patients who are already familiar with exchange lists. Each 15-gram serving is called a "carb choice," and instead of establishing a total number of carbohydrate grams for the day, you will work with your dietitian to determine a total number of carb choices. The following Carb Choices table translates exchanges into carb choices.

▼ CARB CHOICES

Exchange Equivalent	Carb Grams	Carb Choices
1 starch	15 g	1 carb choice
1 fruit	12 g	1 carb choice

Exchange Equivalent	Carb Grams	Carb Choices
3 nonstarchy vegetables	15 g	1 carb choice
1 milk	12 g	1 carb choice
Other carbs	15 g	1 carb choice
Meat	0 g	0 carb choices
Fat	0 g	0 carb choices

Since the choice method involves a certain degree of estimation, this method may not be as exact as calculating carbs strictly by the label. Nonetheless, it is close enough for many people. Talk to your dietitian about the method that works best for you.

Carb counting can also take some practice. In the United States, all food labeling must list carbohydrate content on a per-serving basis, so the carb content in packaged foods is easy to determine. It's important to remember that FDA-prescribed serving sizes and the portions you are used to eating may often be two very different things. Make sure you know how many carbs you are consuming in your serving size and that you account for any extra carbs in bigger servings.

A good carb-counting reference book for fresh whole foods is also a must. Even if you don't cook from scratch, you'll need to know the carb counts in those fruits and veggies, and a carb guide may also be useful for when you're eating out and don't have the benefits of checking labels.

ALERT

When you're planning on enjoying a high-fiber meal or snack, you must adjust your insulin dose accordingly. For any meal with more than 5 grams of fiber, you need to subtract the total fiber from the total carbs before computing your insulin dose.

Advanced Carb Counting

Carbohydrate counting can offer people who use insulin both more control and greater flexibility in what they eat. If you use fast-acting insulin like Humalog or NovoLog prior to a meal, you can determine how many units you need to take based on both your blood sugar reading prior to the meal and on the number of carbohydrate grams you plan to eat. This practice is referred to as "covering" your carbohydrates. The starting point for this "carbohydrate-to-insulin ratio" is about 1:15 (1 unit of insulin for every 15 grams of carbs on the menu). Along with covering the carbohydrates, you should add an additional unit of insulin for every 50 mg/dl that blood sugar is above the target range. For example, if you had 60 grams of carbs on your lunch menu, and your blood sugar levels were 100 mg/dl over your target goal prior to the meal, you would inject 6 units of insulin (4 for the carbs and 2 for the blood sugar). Your mileage may vary; by logging your glucose levels regularly and tracking reactions to meals and insulin, you and your provider should be able to fine-tune your individual ratios.

People who are more insulin resistant may require a larger amount of insulin than those who are more insulin sensitive. Several methods for computing insulin sensitivity exist; and carb-to-insulin ratios are covered elsewhere in this book.

Dietary Exchanges

While most people are now taught carb counting as the method of choice for managing their diabetes, the dietary exchange system is another alternative. It may be preferred by people just learning meal-planning skills, or by those who have difficulty grasping the computations behind carb counting.

The exchange lists are a team effort by the American Diabetes Association and the Academy of Nutrition and Dietetics (formerly the American Dietetic Association), and have been in use for over fifty years. There are three food group types represented in the exchange lists: the carbohydrate group, the meat and meat substitutes group, and the fat group. Each list within each group contains foods with a similar carbohydrate, protein, fat, and calorie content.

When you sit down with your dietitian, she will work with you to specify a certain number of each type of exchanges for your meals, based on your caloric requirements and nutritional needs. You can think of exchanges like trading cards. Any food on a particular list can be swapped with another on the same list. So if you have one fruit exchange allotted for a snack, and you have a taste for fresh fruit instead of the juice you had planned, you could trade your ½ cup of orange juice for 1 cup of raspberries—as both have a roughly equivalent carb, fat, and protein value. Remember that you only trade within lists, not across lists. You can't trade a fruit exchange for a fat exchange, for example.

ESSENTIAL

The exchange lists are based on averages. For whole foods like fruits and vegetables, you'll find the lists to be fairly accurate. Because of variances in food processing and ingredients, you should check the nutritional values of anything you buy with a label to ensure that they are still roughly equivalent to the exchanges you are using.

▼ DIETARY EXCHANGES

	Carbohydrates	Protein	Fat	Calories
Carbohydrate Group				
Starch	15 g	3 g	0–1 g	80
Fruit	15 g	–	–	60
Nonstarchy veggies	5 g	2 g	–	25
Milk, fat-free/low-fat	12 g	8 g	0–3 g	90
Milk, reduced-fat	12 g	8 g	5 g	120
Milk, whole	12 g	8 g	8 g	150
Other carbs (sweets, etc.)	15 g	vary	vary	vary
Meat and Meat Substitutes Group				
Very lean	–	7 g	0–1 g	35
Lean	–	7 g	3 g	55
Medium-fat	–	7 g	5 g	75
High-fat	–	7 g	8 g	100
Fat Group (Oils, Nuts, Etc.)				
All fats	–	–	5 g	45

Some people say they find the exchange system limiting because of the finite number of foods on the "official" exchange lists. Take a walk on the wild side and try something exotic. As long as you have the nutritional breakdown of the food, either on the label or through a food guide or database, you can compute the exchanges yourself. You can also look into purchasing software programs that will help you make the calculations.

Exchanges can also be computed for mixed meals like casseroles, stews, and soups by totaling the carbs, protein, fat, and calories for each ingredient and dividing by the number of servings—the result may be translated into exchanges. You will have to use your measuring tools, however. Cooks who are the "pinch of this, dash of that" type must try to rein in their compulsion and use that food scale. There are dozens of excellent diabetes cookbooks on the market that list full nutritional breakdowns with recipes.

Glycemic Index (GI)

While carbohydrate counting and dietary exchanges are based on the idea that all carbs are created equal and that the total number of carb grams, not the type of carb (i.e., simple or complex, starch or fruit), is the bottom line for blood sugar control, the glycemic index (GI) looks at carb quality instead of quantity.

The GI is a measure of how quickly a carbohydrate affects blood glucose levels. High-GI foods cause quick spikes, while low-GI foods provide a slower, steadier release of glucose. In general, unprocessed, fiber-rich foods tend to be the lowest on the GI scale, while processed and starch-heavy carbohydrates are the highest.

To determine the glycemic index of a food, researchers give a test subject some quantity of the food that contains 50 carbs, and then their blood glucose levels are measured at regular intervals to determine how quickly the carbs in the food turn into glucose. That response is then measured against a standard value of how quickly 50 grams of either glucose or white bread (both 100 on the GI scale) cause blood glucose to rise, which is expressed as a percentage between 1 and 140. The results among a group of testers (usually ten) are averaged to come up with the GI for that food.

Using the GI

Some people with diabetes use the GI as a reference guide to select slow, low-GI carbs in order to keep glucose levels under control and avoid blood sugar spikes. High-GI foods also have their place. If you're about to go for a quick sprint, a pre-exercise carb snack provides the quick release of energy you need. And a fast-acting, high-GI carb is preferable to a low-GI carb for treating hypoglycemia.

ESSENTIAL

Raw foods may have a different GI than the same food cooked, and preparation methods can also impact GI. Fruits may have a lower or higher GI depending on their stage of ripeness. Some foods do not have a GI, and it isn't unusual for the GI of processed foods to vary by brand.

One important caveat when using the GI as your guide: Don't become so carb-centric that you lose sight of your overall nutrient intake. The lower-GI food may not always be the best choice from a nutritional standpoint; a Snickers bar has a GI of 43 while a bowl of Cheerios has a GI of 74. Although this may be your perfect justification for satisfying your sweet tooth, it's obvious that the healthier choice here is the cereal. Keep your vitamin, mineral, protein, and fat intake in perspective.

Glycemic Load

Another anomaly of the GI is that the system doesn't make adjustments for the quantity of carbs per serving. Some foods with a high index value simply don't contain enough carbohydrates per serving to make much of an impact on glucose levels. For example, you'd have to eat more than six servings of cooked beets to get the same amount of carbohydrates from one large baked potato, and yet both of these foods have a relatively high GI (91 and 121, respectively). Researchers at the Harvard School of Public Health have come up with a way to bridge this quality versus quantity gap—the glycemic load. To compute the glycemic load of a food, convert its GI percentage value into decimal format (i.e., 64 is equivalent to 0.64) and multiply it by the grams of carbohydrates in one serving. At first glance, you might want to pass up beets based on their GI alone, despite the fact that they are an excellent source of folate and potassium. But although the GI of cooked beets is 64, a ½-cup serving only has 7 grams of carbs. That makes its glycemic load only 4.48 (0.64 × 7). By comparison, a carb-dense medium baked potato has 27 grams of carbohydrates (with skin), a GI of 69, and a glycemic load of 19.

It's Not Easy

The GI is a good tool for making smart food choices. However, it does require a motivated patient who isn't scared of a little math. And because the GI is not something listed on food labels, it requires a small investment in a book of GI listings. Dr. Jennie Brand-Miller and Dr. Thomas Wolever, two leading authorities on the GI, have coauthored what is arguably the best of the bunch—*The New Glucose Revolution*.

There are also GI databases available online. The Human Nutrition Unit of the University of Sydney is considered the home of the glycemic index. At their website, *www.glycemicindex.com*, you'll find a searchable database of glycemic index and load values for thousands of foods, along with the latest research from Dr. Brand-Miller and her colleagues.

In part because of their relative complexity, the glycemic index and glycemic load have not enjoyed widespread use for diabetes management. But the World Health Organization (WHO) and the European Association for the Study of Diabetes (EASD) have recommended the use of the GI for the nutritional management of diabetes, and the ADA acknowledges that its use "may provide a modest additional benefit over that observed when total carbohydrate is considered alone." If you're interested in trying the GI yourself, talk with your dietitian or doctor about how to incorporate it into your meal plan.

Weights and Measures: Portion Control

You can't measure every morsel that passes your lips, but it's a good idea to measure most foods and beverages until you get a feel for portion sizes. It's a supersized world out there, and most people are surprised to find that their idea of a single serving is actually two or three.

If you're into bells and whistles, there are food scales that are preprogrammed with nutritional information, as well as scales that will keep a running total of your daily food and nutrient intake for you. The only tools you really need, however, are a simple and inexpensive gram scale, dry and liquid measuring cups, and measuring spoons. Early on, it's a good idea to run everything that isn't premeasured through a scale, cup, or spoon first.

Ballparking It

Get intimate with your food, or rather, your dishes. Have a favorite mug or bowl? Pay attention to how completely a serving of yogurt or soup fills it up. You'll soon find that it's second nature to guesstimate your portion sizes. There will be times, however, when you can't use your favorite cup. Pulling out a gram scale at your special restaurant is a little unrealistic. In these cases, it helps to have some rough equivalents for comparison. Here are some typical serving sizes and some points of reference for estimating portion sizes:

- A cup of fruit or yogurt = a baseball, a clenched fist, or a small apple
- Three ounces of fish, meat, or poultry = a deck of cards, the palm of your hand, or a pocket pack of tissues
- One teaspoon of butter or mayonnaise = a thimble, a thumb tip (top knuckle to tip), or the head of a toothbrush
- One ounce of cheese = your entire thumb, a tube of ChapStick, or a AA battery

Using your hands to estimate servings is probably the easiest method—you don't leave home without them. However, make sure you compare your hand amounts against food that has been measured out until you get a sense of how accurately you're estimating. Of course, if you have particularly large or small hands, you need to adjust for size.

FACT

A study published in the *Journal of the American Medical Association* found that over a twenty-one year period, portion sizes of "all-American foods"—salty snacks, desserts, soft drinks, fruit drinks, French fries, hamburgers, cheeseburgers, and Mexican food—grew considerably at fast-food restaurants and at the dinner table. The only exception? Pizza.

Even for the more experienced portion predictor, it's a good idea to test your skills at least once a month and measure your guess at a serving size. It's easy to start overdoing it, and the little bits (and bites) add up. If your control has been off for no apparent reason, one of the first things to check is whether your serving sizes are on target.

Eating Out

Restaurants are notorious for serving up heaping helpings well beyond a single serving size. To keep your intake under control, you can split an entrée, order off the appetizer menu, or simply eat half and take half home. In some restaurants, you may be able to order a child-size portion (but even some children's menu items may be larger than a single serving).

Choosing a Restaurant

When planning a meal out, don't set yourself up for failure. Choose a place that you know offers some food choices that will fit in to your meal plan. Many national restaurant chains, particularly fast-food establishments, will provide nutritional and serving size information on menu items upon request. Ask your server, or look online.

If you must eat at the local greasy spoon—the one that considers lard a food group—fill up on a healthy meal at home first. If you're on the road or in unfamiliar territory, don't be afraid to phone first or ask to see a menu at the door before committing to a restaurant choice. Ask questions about ingredients and preparation method. Explain that you're on a special diet. Some establishments may offer to prepare a dish in an alternate way (e.g., steaming instead of frying it) that isn't on the regular menu.

Smart Ordering

Stay away from the breadbasket, chips and salsa, or other complimentary snacks if you're fond of munching mindlessly. Look for low-carb appetizers on the menu such as antipasto platters, shrimp rémoulade, smoked salmon, and buffalo wings (unbreaded). Cut green veggies with a low-carb dip are also a good option.

ALERT

If you take a before-meal insulin injection, it's a good idea to wait until the food actually arrives at the table before you administer the shot to avoid a blood sugar low. Even if you have the timing down to a science, you never know when slow service or a sudden rush in the kitchen can delay your meal.

Because soda is often dispensed from a fountain at restaurants and bars, it isn't unusual for servers to accidentally substitute regular soda for diet or sugar-free versions. When ordering a diet drink, emphasize the word *diet*. If you're comfortable with doing so, tell your server you have diabetes—wait staff will usually be more mindful of ensuring your order is right if they know your health is at stake. And if you're dining with a large group and are concerned about "look alike" orders being confused with yours, ask for a slice of lemon or lime as a garnish to set your drink or meal apart.

Request that all condiments be served on the side so your food isn't swimming in sauce, and don't be afraid to request reasonable substitutions. If you have a taste for the steak dinner but the stuffed baked potato will be carb overload, ask to swap it for a double serving of the salad or veggies instead.

When Temptation Strikes

You've had a delicious yet healthy meal of broiled fish and steamed veggies and are feeling pleased with yourself for turning down the bacon double-cheeseburger that had been calling your name. And then—the torture device rolls into view, a dessert cart laden with trays of cheesecake, hot fudge cake, and apple-caramel pie. You can feel your blood sugar rising just looking at it.

ESSENTIAL

For some people, diabetes requires a major shift in their perception of food. If you see food as a reward, a comfort when you're feeling down, or a symbol of love for your family, you need to develop positive replacements for it. Food is fuel—look at the quantity and quality of what fills you up analytically rather than emotionally.

You can say "to hell with it!" and order the richest slab of carbs on the dessert cart, or grin and bear it while your dining companion savors his slice of pie à la mode, or use the situation as an opportunity to practice moderation. You will not be struck by lightning if you indulge occasionally, provided your splurges are factored in to your overall meal plan. You can also split a small dessert with a friend, or ask for half now and half in a takeout bag.

If the dessert offerings are truly too rich for your blood, promise yourself a favorite low-carb treat on your way home. Don't deny yourself—it's not an all-or-nothing game. In fact, the stress of constantly doing so may raise your blood glucose levels higher than the occasional brownie.

Social occasions centered around eating, such as birthday parties, holiday gatherings, or family reunion barbecues, offer you a whole new set of challenges. You might find that well-meaning friends and relatives feel the need to be the food police, asking with every pass of the plate, "Should you be eating that?" The best answer is simple: "Most people with diabetes can eat just about anything you can, in moderation. I have a few books you can borrow that explain more if you're interested." With any luck, they'll take you up on your offer and learn a thing or two. If they don't, you've probably stopped them from pestering you, at least until Thanksgiving.

Smart Snack Substitutes

Even though you can indulge occasionally, if you've made a regular habit of junk food, it's a habit you'll have to kick. Still, having many small meals, or minisnacks between meals, can be beneficial to keeping blood glucose on an even keel. Your RD will work these in to your meal plan.

Cut out the fatty fried snacks, sugary drinks and sodas, and sugar-crusted snack pies. Instead, try some of these healthier snack choices; all have around 15 grams of carbs (one carb choice) or fewer:

- Air-popped popcorn (3 cups)
- Snack-size sugar-free Jell-O with Cool Whip (both are free exchanges)
- Five whole-wheat crackers with peanut butter (1 tablespoon)
- Sugar-free pudding (½ cup)
- Two small tangerines
- Baked tortilla chips (15 to 20) and salsa

Regaining Control after a Fall

If you haven't already, at one point in your life you will probably end up with an "Oh, wow!" reading after splurging on something you shouldn't have. Ask yourself if there was a specific trigger for the slip-up. Maybe you had a particularly stressful day at work or went to a party hungry. If you can pinpoint a cause, think about how you can prevent it from happening next time, whether by adjusting your eating schedule or learning some stress management techniques.

It is not the end of the world if you slip up. If you're too busy kicking yourself for your mistake, you'll miss any lesson you might gain. Diabetes is a disease of highs and lows, both physically and emotionally. Strive to achieve balance in the emotional area as well as the physical one.

Blood Sugar Savers

You probably know the usual suspects when it comes to foods that will raise your blood sugar. Sugar-rich desserts, potatoes, pastries, pasta, breads . . . the list goes on and on. But did you know that some foods can actually help even out those blood sugar spikes? Pack your pantry with these blood sugar savers and start working them into your daily meal plan.

Vinegar and Fermented Foods

The acetic acid in vinegar moderates blood sugar response and also contributes to a feeling of fullness following a meal, which may in turn cause you to eat less. This also holds true for fermented foods like olives, sauerkraut, kimchi, and pickles (which are not technically fermented, but pickled in vinegar brine).

FACT

Love bread but hate the rise in blood sugar it causes? Try sourdough bread. Unlike yeast-based breads, sourdough is made through a fermented leavening process, with a dough that contains lactic acid. This acidic substance is the reason that sourdough causes a significantly lower blood sugar rise than nonsourdough breads.

Dressing salads or veggies with oil and vinegar is an easy way to work vinegar into your dietary repertoire. To increase the effect, add a little lemon juice to the mix, which also moderates blood sugar with its high acidity. You can marinate proteins like fish, beef, and chicken in a vinegar mixture as well. There are many flavors and varieties of vinegar to choose from; if you choose a vinaigrette or a fruit-based vinegar, be sure to check the total carbohydrates on the label to make sure you aren't canceling out the benefits of this versatile condiment.

Nuts

The good monounsaturated fatty acids in nuts have proven benefits to heart health and improvements in cholesterol levels. Nuts can also help level out blood sugar spikes when eaten with carb-rich foods. The protein and fats, and possibly the phytochemicals, in tree nuts help mediate the post-prandial (after-meal) blood sugar response to carb-rich foods. Their high fiber content may also add to a feeling of fullness, which can be beneficial if you are trying to lose weight.

So throw a handful of almonds in your salad, add peanuts to a stir fry, or sprinkle slivered nuts on your favorite fish or chicken dish. Although nuts are nutrient dense, they are also calorie dense, so keep portions small.

Cinnamon

Studies have had conflicting results as to whether or not cinnamon can help lower your blood sugar levels. Most animal studies have shown a benefit, while human studies have been less conclusive. However, a 2012 meta-analysis published in *The American Journal of Clinical Nutrition* found that cinnamon had beneficial effects on both fasting blood sugar levels and A1C, at least up to four months of use. Cinnamon intake for this study ranged between one and six grams daily, which is a lot of cinnamon.

More research on this spice is needed to develop better guidelines on how much cinnamon is helpful. In the meantime, an extra sprinkle in your coffee, yogurt, fruit, and other cinnamon-friendly foods certainly can't hurt you, and might even help.

CHAPTER 6

Get Active . . . Get Healthy!

One of the simplest and most effective ways to bring down blood sugar levels, cut the risk of cardiovascular disease, and improve overall health and well-being is exercise. Despite these benefits, exercise is a tough sell in our increasingly sedentary world where almost every essential task can be performed online, from the driver's seat, or with a phone call. Redefining your preconceived notions of exercise, and making it fun, is the best way to ensure that you look forward to exercising instead of finding ways to avoid it.

The Importance of Exercise

Everyone should exercise, yet the National Health Interview Survey tells us that less than half of the U.S. adult population gets the recommended thirty minutes of daily physical activity—and 33 percent aren't active at all. Inactivity is thought to be one of the key reasons for the surge of type 2 diabetes in the United States, because inactivity and obesity promote insulin resistance.

The good news is that it's never too late to get moving, and exercise is one of the easiest ways to start controlling your diabetes. Exercise can improve insulin sensitivity, lower the risk of heart disease, and promote weight loss. For people with type 2 diabetes, studies have demonstrated that regular exercise can lower A1C levels, reduce cardiovascular risk, and promote weight loss. Regular structured exercise of eight weeks or more lowers A1C values by an average of 0.66 percent in this population.

In 2011, the American Diabetes Association and the American College of Sports Medicine released joint exercise guidelines for people with type 2 diabetes. The guidelines recommend a minimum of 150 minutes of moderate intensity aerobic exercise weekly, spread out over at least three days each week. Ideally, no more than two days should pass between aerobic exercise sessions. In addition to aerobic activity, resistance training is also recommended two to three times a week, except for individuals who have other health conditions or complications that make resistance exercise unadvisable.

FACT

Resistance training is strength training that works the muscles. Activities such as weight lifting, working with resistance bands, water workouts, and body weight resistance exercises (e.g., push ups or pull ups) are all good forms of resistance training.

Getting Started

The first order of business with any exercise plan, especially if you're a dyed-in-the-wool couch potato, is to consult with your health care provider. If you have cardiac risk factors, she may want to perform a stress test to establish a safe level of exercise for you.

Certain diabetic complications also dictate what type of exercise program you can take on. For people with diabetic retinopathy, activities like weightlifting, jogging, or high-impact aerobics may pose a risk for further blood vessel damage and possible retinal detachment. Patients with severe peripheral neuropathy (PN) may need to avoid foot-intensive weight-bearing exercises such as long-distance walking, jogging, or step aerobics and opt instead for low-impact activities like swimming, biking, and rowing. If you have conditions that make exercise a challenge, your care provider may refer you to an exercise physiologist who can design a fitness program for your specific needs.

The good news is that no matter what your fitness level or related diabetic complications may be, a physical activity program can be tailored to work for you. And as you start to benefit from the health improvements that come along with regular exercise, you may be able to ramp up your physical activity level under the guidance of your health care provider.

If you're already active in sports or work out regularly, you will still benefit from a discussion with your doctor about your regular exercise routine. If you're taking insulin, you may need to take special precautions to prevent both hypoglycemia and hyperglycemia during or after your workout.

Start Slowly

Your exercise routine can be as simple as a brisk nightly neighborhood walk. If you haven't been very active before now, start slowly and work your way up. Walk the dog or get out in the yard and rake. Take the stairs instead of the elevator. Park in the back of the lot and walk. Every little bit does, in fact, help.

ALERT

Leg pain during exercise that goes away with rest, especially aching in the calves, buttocks, or thighs, could be a sign of intermittent claudication and peripheral vascular disease (a potential complication of diabetes). Physician-supervised exercise, particularly walking, can actually help ease the pain over time. Medication may also be required.

As little as thirty minutes of daily, heart-pumping exercise can make a big difference in improving your blood sugar control and reducing your risk of developing diabetic complications. One of the easiest and least expensive ways of getting moving is to start a walking program. All you need is a good pair of well-fitting, supportive shoes and a direction to head in.

Do pay particular attention to your feet both before and after you walk or run. Because of the risk for foot ulcers and other diabetic foot problems, you should examine your feet carefully for blisters and abrasions, and then treat them promptly if they do occur. Seamless, waterproof socks that wick moisture away from your feet can help to prevent friction while walking.

Making Time

Everyone is busy. But considering what's at stake, making time for exercise needs to be a priority right now. Thirty minutes a day isn't much time when you get right down to it. Cut one primetime show out of your evening television-viewing schedule. Get up a half-hour earlier each morning. Use half of your lunch hour for a brisk walk. You can find the time if you look hard enough for it.

You can also try combining exercise with something else already on your schedule. If you normally spend an hour on Saturday mornings playing video games with your kids, take the game out of the virtual world and play a real game of touch football or Frisbee outside. Get off the riding mower and cut the grass the old-fashioned way—with a manual push mower. Wake up early and walk your kids to school. Look for opportunities rather than excuses.

Exercise Intensity

How hard you should push yourself during exercise depends on your level of fitness and your health history. Your doctor can recommend an optimal heart rate target for working out based on those factors. It's very important to get this information from your doctor before starting an exercise program, especially if you have a history of cardiovascular problems.

On average, most people should aim for a target heart rate zone of 50 to 75 percent of their maximum heart rate. Maximum heart rate is computed by subtracting your age from the number 220. So, if you are 40, your maximum heart rate would be 180, and your target heart rate zone would be between 90 and 135 beats per minute.

You should wear a digital or analog watch with a second hand or function to check your heart rate during exercise. To calculate your heart rate, place your fingers at your wrist or neck pulse point and count the number of beats for fifteen seconds. Multiply that number by four to get your heart rate. The number you get should be within your target zone. If it's too high, take your intensity down a few notches. If you're exercising below your target zone, pick things up. If you are new to exercise, you should aim for the lower (50 percent) range of your target heart rate. As you become more fit, you can work toward the 75 percent maximum.

Blood Sugars and Exercise

When you exercise, your body uses glucose for energy. During the first fifteen minutes of your workout routine, your body converts the glycogen stored in your muscles back into glucose, and also uses the glucose circulating in your bloodstream for fuel, lowering blood sugar levels. At the same time, the body produces some counter-regulatory hormones, such as adrenalin, during a workout. These can cause blood sugar to rise following exercise. The natural blood-sugar-regulating effects of exercise can last up to twenty-four hours, so it's important to test your blood sugar not just before and during exercise, but afterward as well.

FACT

The type 2 diabetes drugs glyburide, glipizide, glimepiride, nateglinide, and repaglinide are all considered insulin secretagogues. These diabetes drugs work by triggering the release of insulin by the pancreas. People who take these drugs are at risk for hypoglycemia episodes.

People who are on insulin or other diabetes drugs that trigger the release of insulin in the body (known as *insulin secretagogues*) have a risk of hypoglycemia during and after exercise. If you take one of these drugs, you should always test your blood sugar levels before you get moving. If your levels are less than 100 mg/dl, you may not want to start working out without first eating a carbohydrate snack for fuel. A fast-acting carb should be available during and after your workout, in case you need it.

Snacking Savvy

If you take insulin or another diabetes medicine that puts you at risk for low blood sugar episodes, you may need to eat a pre-exercise snack prior to your workout. How much of a snack and when to eat it depends on your blood sugar readings and the planned intensity and duration of your workout.

If your blood sugar is below 100 mg/dl, you should consider having 15 g of carbohydrates before starting exercise. Adding protein and/or fat to the carbs can extend the glucose action over time, which is important if you're embarking on a long-distance bike ride or similar activity. The snack should be eaten about fifteen to thirty minutes before exercise for the best results.

If you're going on a low-intensity, half-hour walk and your glucose readings are at least 100 mg/dl, you may not need any extra carbs (although you should always bring some with you just in case).

ALERT

If you have blood sugars greater than 300 mg/dl (without the presence of ketones on a blood or urine test), you can still engage in exercise provided you feel well and drink plenty of fluids to stay well-hydrated. If your levels are high and you do choose to exercise, make sure you test blood sugar levels again about fifteen minutes into your workout to ensure they are coming back down.

Be wary of exercise immediately following an insulin injection. Give your body time—at least ninety minutes—to digest and process injected insulin. Don't plan exercise during the time your insulin is peaking. Exercise can also cause injected insulin to work much faster because your circulation speeds up as your heart pumps harder. In many cases, you may need to adjust your insulin dose downward for those times you will be exercising; again, your doctor can offer you further advice on what's right for you.

Lows (Hypoglycemia)

If you start to feel hypoglycemia coming on, don't panic. Stop exercising and test immediately. If your levels are too low, eat or drink 15 grams of simple carbohydrate right away. Don't resume your workout. Wait fifteen minutes for the carbs to kick in and test again. If your levels are still too low, take 15 more grams and follow the same routine until blood glucose levels are back in a normal range. A glucose gel or glucose tablet is a good choice for a fast-acting carb. Both are compact enough to carry along with you while you exercise and work quickly. Invest in a waterproof fanny pack to carry both your glucose gel/tablets and testing supplies during your workout.

After your workout is finished, your body will recharge its energy stores by processing your blood glucose into glycogen. Depending on the level of exercise intensity and the amount of glycogen that needs to be replaced, this process could take anywhere from four to twenty-four hours. This is why postexercise blood sugar testing is important, as hypoglycemia can occur well after you've finished exercising.

ESSENTIAL

Keeping an exercise log along with your blood glucose readings can help you figure out what works best for you. Different sports and routines will have diverse effects on your blood sugar levels. Discuss your exercise plans with your diabetes care team to find out the best routine for preparing for exercise.

To avoid dangerous highs and lows during exercise, take the following precautions:

- **Test first.** Always take a blood glucose reading before your workout.
- **Warm up.** Always stretch out before exercising to avoid injury, and start your routine with five to ten minutes of low-intensity movement.
- **Wet down.** Drink plenty of fluids before, during, and after your workout to prevent dehydration. If you're exercising in the heat, drink even more. (Be aware that many exercise and energy drinks contain high amounts of carbohydrates.)

- **Cool off.** If you're working out intensely, take it down a few notches at a time, and spend five to ten minutes bringing your heart rate back down to its preworkout level.
- **Carb load.** Have a fast-acting carbohydrate on hand in case of hypoglycemia, and don't hesitate to use it.
- **Test last.** Once your workout is over, test your blood glucose levels again to ensure they aren't dipping too low.

Everyone Can Exercise

Virtually anyone who has the capability to move can exercise to some degree. Even if you suffer from complications related to your diabetes or other health conditions, your doctor can recommend a level and form of exercise that is appropriate for you.

Chances are that you already work out without even knowing it. Activities that you have never considered "exercise," like washing the car or cleaning your house, are actually calorie-burning, heart-pumping ways to get fit. According to the U.S. Surgeon General, all of the following activities will burn about 150 calories a day (or 1,000 calories a week):

- Washing and waxing a car for 45 to 60 minutes
- Washing windows or floors for 45 to 60 minutes
- Gardening for 30 to 45 minutes
- Pushing a stroller 1.5 miles in 30 minutes
- Raking leaves for 30 minutes
- Walking 2 miles in 30 minutes (15 minutes per mile)
- Doing water aerobics for 30 minutes
- Bicycling 4 miles in 15 minutes
- Shoveling snow for 15 minutes
- Climbing steps for 15 minutes

Disabled and Chronically Ill

For people with orthopedic conditions, joint pain, or musculoskeletal problems, low-impact exercise is usually the best bet. Swimming is a good low-impact form of resistance exercise. If you are in a wheelchair or unable to stand or stay on your feet for long periods without support, chair exercises may also be a good option. There are a number of chair-exercise DVDs available for home workouts.

Dealing with Obesity

If you are extremely overweight or obese, exercise is especially important yet can present unique challenges. Comfort is an issue; certain exercises like jogging and high-impact aerobics may simply not be feasible. Weight lies heavy on the mind as well as the body, and it's possible you may not feel mentally or emotionally prepared to join group or team exercises.

The solution is to work on your own level. Don't try step aerobics just yet. Contact your local YMCA or community center to see if there's a plus-size exercise program available. And always check with your doctor before starting a new fitness routine. A referral to an exercise physiologist may be appropriate, particularly if you have other health problems.

It may be easier said than done, but don't feel self-conscious. If you feel uncomfortable amid all the spandex and ripped abs at the local health club, then don't torture yourself—find an environment that you feel comfortable in. Try a walking program, either outside or at home on a treadmill. The impact-free environment of a pool is also a good place to start getting fit. Buddy up with a friend and motivate each other to reach workout goals. Exercise should make you feel good about yourself. Every step you take is a step toward a healthier you.

QUESTION

I have trouble walking and am confined to a wheelchair. Do I have any exercise options?
Absolutely. Even if you can't use your lower body, it's important to keep your upper body active and toned to get all the health benefits of regular exercise. There are plenty of exercises that can be done seated, including lifting light weights and using resistance bands. Speak with your doctor first to get medical clearance, and then consider seeing an exercise physiologist who can help you design a workout from your wheelchair.

Exercising for the Elderly

Staying active is particularly important as you grow older. Aging is associated with increased insulin resistance, and it's thought that this is at least partially attributable to a loss of muscle mass. Keep on track with an active lifestyle and strength-training exercises to retain muscle mass and insulin sensitivity. It's never too late to get moving. Talk to your doctor today about an appropriate exercise program that promotes strength, balance, flexibility, and endurance.

Get Your Kids to Exercise, Too

Obviously, exercise is good for everyone in your family, kids included. For overweight children, or adolescents with type 2 diabetes, or those who are considered at risk for the disease, exercise is absolutely imperative for all the reasons previously cited for adults: weight loss, improved insulin sensitivity, and overall health and well-being.

And of course, if you are reading this because you have type 2 diabetes, your family history means that your kids are at increased risk for the disease. Instilling healthy physical activity habits early in life is important. So plan regular activities that involve the whole family. From family hikes to scavenger hunts, there are many creative ways to get kids moving.

Staying Motivated

One of the biggest obstacles to staying on track for fitness is losing motivation. People who are just starting an exercise program can quickly become tired of the same routine, day after day. Keeping exercise appealing and maintaining a good fitness perspective is key to staying motivated and to the long-term success of your fitness program.

Boredom Busters

If you had to watch the same exact episode of your favorite television show every day for the rest of your life, you'd probably be banging your head against the wall by the end of the week. You'd change the channel, pick up a book, or do anything you could to avoid something you once enjoyed. Yet many people starting on a fitness program feel compelled to follow the same routine, day after day after day, and consequently fall off the exercise wagon due to sheer boredom. Try these strategies to keep your workouts interesting:

- **Mix and match.** Play racquetball with a friend one week, and then try water polo the next.
- **Buddy up.** Get a walking partner or an exercise buddy to keep you motivated (and vice versa).
- **Join a team.** Find a local softball league or aerobics group. Even when you aren't feeling much like exercising, your commitment to other team members may get you moving.
- **Relocate.** If you like to bike, walk, or jog, try a new route or locale.
- **Go for the goal.** Set new fitness targets for yourself.
- **Reward yourself.** When you reach a new goal, pat yourself on the back with a nonedible reward.
- **Make some noise.** Forget the radio and your CDs and customize your own soundtrack for working out.
- **Be well read.** Exercise your mind as well as your body with an audiobook.
- **Sound off.** Try exercising without the iPod for once, and enjoy the sounds of nature and the neighborhood.

Keeping It in Perspective

Many people with type 2 diabetes start exercising for the sole purpose of losing weight. When the pounds don't drop as quickly or as completely as they'd like, some of these people get discouraged and give up. If you take away any message about exercise and diabetes, let it be this: Even if you don't lose weight, your investment in exercise is still paying off in reduced heart disease risk and better blood sugar control. Also, remember exercise builds muscle, which weighs more than fat. So if your clothes fit better, but the pounds don't melt off as much as you hope— you are still ahead of the game. And exercise simply makes you feel better, both physically and mentally. Your energy level will rise and the endorphins released by your brain during exercise will boost your sense of well-being and may help fight diabetes-related depression. Don't give up before you really get started. You owe it to yourself to keep going.

CHAPTER 7

Testing Your Blood Sugar

A home blood glucose monitor—a device that analyzes a blood sample and gives you a reading of your current blood sugar levels—is the next best thing to having a lab in your medicine cabinet. Monitors (also called meters) are probably the single, most useful tool you have for knowing what's going on with your diabetes, mainly because they are always accessible, provide instant results, and don't require a trip to the doctor's office.

Why Test?

Regular self-monitoring of blood glucose levels (SMBG) gives you a quick clinical snapshot of exactly where your blood glucose levels are at any given moment. Testing, and keeping a detailed log of test results and the circumstances that surround them, will help you understand how certain foods and activities affect your blood sugar. Once you are able to detect patterns in blood glucose changes over time, you can use the information to adjust your treatment accordingly.

Another role of SMBG is to help you assess how effective your medication or insulin is in controlling your glucose levels. SMBG is also an invaluable tool for adjusting the timing of medication to ensure the best possible control.

QUESTION

I can't stand the thought of sticking myself. Can't I just test for sugar in my urine?
You could, but it would do little to help you control your diabetes. Because urine collects in your bladder for several hours before it leaves the body and only contains glucose when blood levels are over 180 mg/dl, it isn't a very timely or sensitive test. Worse, it cannot help detect potentially dangerous low blood sugar levels.

Most important, SMBG can help you avoid life-threatening blood sugar emergencies. If you are under stress, sick with the flu, or taking medications that affect blood glucose levels, regular testing can help you keep close tabs on your blood sugar levels so you can take action before they go dangerously high.

Testing before, after, and possibly during exercise can help you avoid a precipitous drop in blood sugar levels. It's also wise to test if you've been drinking alcohol, another trigger for hypoglycemia. If you feel a low coming on, a quick test can confirm your levels so you can take immediate action.

Developing a Testing Schedule

When to test is a matter of debate. Some people test once when they wake up. Others test many more times a day—morning, night, and before and after meals. As a general rule, when your diagnosis is new and you're learning how different factors affect your diabetes, you should check your blood sugar levels frequently.

The same holds true for monitoring any changes to your treatment routine. SMBG can help you and your doctor assess how medication and other changes are working to improve your diabetes control.

ALERT

If you suspect a blood sugar low, you should always test yourself immediately. Treat yourself with 15 grams of fast-acting carbohydrate, (or more based on how low your blood sugar may be) wait fifteen minutes, and then test again. If blood sugars are still not in a safe range, repeat the process. If your meter isn't around but you feel low, treat it first and test later.

When to Test

The ADA recommends that people with type 2 diabetes who are on multiple insulin injection therapy or use insulin pumps test three or more times daily. There are no specific ADA recommendations for frequency of testing in patients who aren't on insulin, or for those who are on once or twice daily insulin injections. But again, self-monitoring is the best available tool to provide immediate feedback on how food, exercise, medication, and other environmental factors are affecting your blood sugars.

FACT

In the United States, home blood glucose monitors display readings as mg/dl (milligrams over deciliters). However, everywhere outside the United States, the standard is mmol/l (millimoles over liters). Some monitors that are sold internationally may have an option for switching back and forth between mg/dl and mmol/l displays.

Although the cost of testing supplies can sometimes be a barrier, self-monitoring should be performed as frequently as possible to help achieve blood sugar goals. Postprandial, or after-meal, testing is also encouraged at two hours after the start of meal. Testing after eating allows you to see how different foods and food combinations impact your blood sugar levels, and will also reveal trends that can help you to bring down a high A1C.

Overcoming Testing Barriers

It's natural for you to have some hesitation about sticking yourself on a regular basis. But it's important to realize that today's lancets, the needle-like devices used to prick your finger to obtain a blood sample, are extremely fine, easy to use, and virtually painless. Your diabetes educator can show you simple methods for drawing an adequate blood sample with minimal discomfort.

As mentioned, cost can have an impact on how frequently you can test. When determining a schedule for blood sugar testing with your doctor, make sure you discuss any financial or insurance issues that may affect your testing routine. Test strips are expensive (a package will likely cost more than the monitor itself), and most insurance plans have a preferred test strip brand, which will typically be the least expensive brand. Some plans may put a cap on the quantity of testing supplies they will cover for a given time period. Find out what your insurer offers and work from there. In some cases, your provider may be able to offer you some free product samples to augment your supply.

Target Goals

Your ultimate goal is to get your blood sugar levels as close to normal as possible. However, if you have medical conditions that affect your control, your target glucose levels may need to be kept a bit higher. A newly diagnosed child or adolescent with diabetes who may not yet have the ability to recognize symptoms of hypoglycemia also may have higher goals. You should work with your doctor to establish self-monitoring goals that are right for you.

▼ **GENERAL GUIDELINES FOR AVERAGE TARGET BLOOD SUGAR LEVELS**

Test Time	ADA Guideline	AACE Guideline
Preprandial (fasting or before meals)	70–130 mg/dl (3.9–7.2 mmol/l)	<110 mg/dl (6.1 mmol/l)
Postprandial (1 to 2 hours after start of meal)	<180 mg/dl (10.0 mmol/l) at 1 to 2 hours	<140 mg/dl at two hours (7.8 mmol/l)

The Blood Sugar Meter and Other Equipment

Your first order of business is choosing a monitor that's accurate, easy to use, and comfortable. In some cases, your insurance plan may dictate the brand or type you get. If you have some latitude in selecting a meter, be sure to ask for recommendations. Your diabetes educator, members of your support group, your pharmacist, and your physician are all good sources.

The U.S. Food and Drug Administration (FDA) regulations for the manufacture of blood glucose monitors suggest that monitors be accurate within 20 percent of laboratory reference values. That may seem like a lot of variance, but as long as your meter is consistent in its readings and you know how much it differs from laboratory values (which your doctor can help you determine), the variance isn't too critical. If a reading seems excessively high or low, try testing again.

Anatomy of a Meter

Blood glucose monitors come in all shapes and sizes, but there are some common features that most share:

- **Display.** Blood glucose readings are digitally displayed on a small screen in blood plasma values of mg/dl (milligrams over deciliter). The screen will also display error codes and instructions on calibration.
- **Buttons and beepers.** The operator's manual for your monitor will explain the button functions. Your meter may also have special audio signals to let you know when a test is complete or to alert you of highs and lows.
- **Test strip slot.** Your blood sample goes on a test strip, which is inserted into the meter. Some meters use self-enclosed test-strip drums or cartridges, which are automatically fed into the meter, so the user does not have to handle the strip.
- **Memory.** Most modern meters have some type of memory feature that can record a predetermined number of glucose readings. Some meters will also let you mark readings taken around insulin doses and generate different average glucose readings.

- **Battery.** Meters are battery powered, and many have a warning system that will tell you when the battery power starts to get low. It's a good idea to keep an extra set of batteries on hand for backup.

Other bells and whistles you may find on your glucose monitor include larger displays or voice modules for patients with vision problems, backlit displays or glow-in-the-dark cases and skins for easy night testing, and computer compatibility for downloading glucose data to special software programs or even to wireless devices. New meter technology can wirelessly transmit testing data to insulin pumps and recognize and alert you to testing trends.

In 2012, the first home glucose monitor that integrates with a smartphone was introduced in the U.S. market. The iBGStar (Sanofi) is a small testing unit that plugs into an iPhone or iPod Touch device. A test strip is inserted into the unit and blood sugar readings are stored right on the iPhone or iPod device with a diabetes management app that can also track insulin, carb intake, and any patterns in blood sugar control.

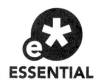

ESSENTIAL

Bring your blood glucose meter along with you to your doctor's appointments. If you're new to testing, or you're using a new brand of meter, your physician can compare the readings with laboratory values to ensure accuracy. In addition, your doctor may want to see your testing technique when you review your self-management.

There are a growing number of meters on the market that do more than just test blood sugar levels. Some combine technologies to also test ketones or blood pressure with a single device. These multitasking meters may be a good choice if you want to cut down on your clutter.

Obtaining the Blood Sample

You draw the blood for testing with a lancet, which is a small, fine needle. Lancets come in a small plastic case. They can be used alone or inserted into a spring-loaded lancing device, which quickly pierces the skin at a preset depth.

Lancets are available in different gauges (e.g., 21 gauge, 30 gauge)—the higher the gauge, the sharper the lancet, and the smaller the insertion hole at the test site. A higher-gauge lancet will, theoretically, make for a less painful stick (although factors such as skin sensitivity and test site factor in, too). High-gauge lancets may also be preferable for children.

Many monitors come with a separate lancing pen, while others have a lancing device integrated into the monitor itself. Lancing devices can also be purchased separately. Most spring-loaded lancing devices allow the user to set the depth of the lancet stick. Calloused skin may require a deeper stick, while a more shallow lancet stick may be better suited to sensitive skin.

Most lancet manufacturers recommend using a fresh lancet with each test. Their rationale is that each use damages the needle slightly and makes subsequent tests more painful. However, in practice people with diabetes often wait a day or even a week to swap out lancets to save money and time, and reduce waste. Whatever you choose to do, never share your lancing device with another person; and if testing gets more painful, try using a fresh lancet.

The lancets you use depend on three factors:

1. The requirements of the lancet device provider with your meter
2. The sensitivity and condition of your fingers (for instance, calloused fingers may require thicker lancets)
3. The size of the blood sample required—some meters only require a blood drop as small as a pinhead

Alternative Site Testing

To the relief of sore fingers everywhere, there are glucose monitors available that allow testing on less sensitive parts of the body, such as the forearm or thigh. These alternative site meters may be a good choice for you if you have sensitive fingers, and you find yourself testing less frequently because of it.

However, be aware that test results from alternative sites of the body can vary from fingertip testing. Blood drawn from the fingertips may register glucose changes in the body faster than blood drawn from other testing sites.

The FDA has required alternative site meter manufacturers to label their products with this information. If you are experiencing signs of hypoglycemia, or if you have hypoglycemic unawareness, always test from your fingertips to ensure the most accurate readings.

Test Strips

A test strip is a small rectangular piece of chemically treated paper or plastic that collects your blood sample for analysis by your monitor. Most meters require that you insert a new strip for each test. However, some strips designed for specific meters come in self-contained "drums" that change the strip for you with each use.

Additionally, some test strips have special control codes that the meter must be calibrated against. Depending on the type of blood glucose meter you own, you may have to code your meter each time you open a new package of test strips. This process is typically fairly quick and simple.

ESSENTIAL

Extreme temperature swings can affect the accuracy of meters and test strips. For this reason, avoid stowing your meter and supplies in your car in hot or cold weather, and don't leave your equipment outside in direct sunlight or extreme cold.

The accuracy of your blood tests depends on the quality and treatment of your test strips, so don't gamble with your health by cutting corners. Using expired strips is dangerous, because they may not be able to detect your glucose levels accurately. Test strips are costly, and buying strips in large quantities is usually cheaper than the smaller-quantity packages. However, if you end up with half-used containers of strips and have to throw them away, then you haven't saved anything.

Many third-party manufacturers (companies that manufacture strips compatible with other manufacturers' brands of meters) produce strips for use in a variety of meter makes and models. These third-party strips can often be less expensive than the brand name strips. However, you need to be sure that the third-party strips have been tested for use with your specific monitor. The test strip package labeling and directions for use should list this information. If you don't see your monitor make and model listed, don't buy the strips. Your monitor manufacturer often can provide you with a list of compatible third-party test strips.

Always keep your test strips out of excessive heat and moisture. The bathroom is a poor choice for storage, as humidity can affect strip accuracy. Storing your strips inside of your meter case in their original package will ensure that they stay clean.

Accessorize!

Stuffing your meter in a back pocket or letting it float around in the bottom of your purse with ATM receipts, broken breath mints, and other assorted junk isn't a good idea. You trust your health to this piece of equipment, so treat it carefully. Many meters come with a carrying case for protection—use it. If your meter didn't come with a case, a well-padded cosmetic bag, shaving kit, or similar container will do the trick, too. There are also plenty of stylish meter cases available for sale in a variety of shapes and sizes.

Your test strips and control solution also need to be kept clean, dry, and at room temperature. Keep them in the case with your monitor and lancing supplies, and you'll have everything properly stored and together when you need it.

How It Works

So, how do you test? First, read the instructions that come with your meter. Even if you're a "do first, ask for directions later" kind of a person, stifle that instinct. Every meter operates a little differently, and you may be required to perform calibration procedures, or other steps, that are outlined in the directions for use.

Glucose testing involves using a lancet to prick your fingertip (or other area of your body) to get a blood sample. When performed on the finger, this process is called a finger stick. The blood drop that comes out of the finger stick is then placed on a test strip that has been inserted into the glucose meter. Many meters feature strips that actually draw in or absorb the blood sample.

Once the meter detects an adequate sample of blood on the strip, it will measure the amount of glucose present, and then display the results on the screen in either an mg/dl or mmol/l reading. Some meters will display special alarms or warnings if the readings are excessively high or low. Getting results can take anywhere from a few seconds to a minute, but the majority of new meters display results in ten seconds or less.

Following are some tips to improve the ease, accuracy, and usefulness of your testing:

- **Wash your hands thoroughly.** Any food, medication residue, or other substances on your fingers can affect test results. Even hand lotion can contain sugars that could falsely raise your test numbers. Make sure your testing site is dry, as water can dilute the blood sample and give you a falsely low value.
- **If you use rubbing alcohol on the test site, let it dry before lancing.** Some people choose to disinfect their skin with an alcohol swab before testing. Pricking the skin before the alcohol dries can cause stinging or burning.
- **Experiment with different gauge lancets.** The thickness, or gauge, of your lancet affects both the size of the blood sample and how painful it feels.
- **Experiment with different lancet depths.** Spring-loaded lancing devices often offer an option for adjusting how far into the skin the needle pierces.
- **Get the blood flowing to your hands before you stick yourself.** If you have problems getting an adequate drop of blood, you can stimulate circulation by running your hands under warm water, rubbing them together, or shaking them at your sides.
- **Stick the sides of your fingers.** The pad of your finger is more sensitive and therefore more painful to stick, so try lancing the side of your fingertip instead.

Troubleshooting

Even with the most fastidious testing methods, sometimes the numbers just won't seem right. If you think your technique may be to blame, review the operator's manual and test again. Certain medical conditions (such as anemia) and substances (such as vitamin C) can influence glucose testing results. Talk with your doctor if you have coexisting medical conditions or if you are taking other medications or supplements outside of your diabetes drugs.

Quality Control

If your readings are off, you may be able to use the quality-control tools that are part of your meter kit. Control solution is a glucose-based liquid that is used in place of blood to ensure your meter is working correctly. If the reading on your meter matches the range of values on the control solution label, then your meter should be providing accurate readings. Your meter may also include a special electronic control strip that is used to ensure that the meter is operating properly. Read your meter instructions to find out more on how and when to use these features.

QUESTION

Why does my meter have such different results than my doctor's equipment?
The U.S. FDA allows for home blood glucose meters to be as much as 15 to 20 percent lower or higher than laboratory standards, which may explain the variance. Get to know your particular meter and how it trends. If the numbers seem very wrong, try a different meter.

Calibration

Many glucose monitors must be calibrated for use with your test strips before use. Test strips will be labeled with a number that must be entered into the meter. Check both your owner's manual and test strip documentation for information on calibrating test strip type. If your strips are calibrated correctly and the readings still seem to be off, try one from a new package (and report problems with the old package to the strip manufacturer).

Keep It Clean

A dirty meter or dirty, damaged test strips can give false readings. The instructions for use that came with your glucose monitor should tell you how and when to clean it. Be aware that some monitors are not designed to be cleaned, so always read the directions first.

Wear and Tear

Even the most rugged meters will wear out eventually. If you're getting frequent error codes or your monitor is giving erratic readings, it may just be time to trade in your trusty old friend for a newer model.

Tracking Your Test Results

Your test results are most useful if you view them in the context of the rest of your day. Log your readings, along with your medications, insulin, food intake, exercise, and other significant events. Over time, patterns will emerge, and you will probably discover certain triggers that make your blood glucose levels fluctuate. Your doctor and diabetes educator can help you interpret the data further.

Some glucose monitors have memory features that allow you to store several weeks' or even months' worth of readings, compute averages, and indicate which readings occurred in conjunction with an insulin shot, eating, or activities like exercise. These readings can also be helpful in detecting patterns.

Logbooks

Many monitors come with a logbook for recording the results, but a notebook will do the job just as well. When recording your readings, make sure you note the time of the test (i.e., preprandial/postprandial) and the time and amount of medication and/or insulin taken. For an even more complete picture of what's happening with your blood glucose levels, you can also note what you eat at each meal.

The sample logbook shown that follows includes entry spaces for before-meal (preprandial) and after-meal (postprandial) blood glucose results, plus a space to record the carbs consumed in each meal and the accompanying insulin dose or mixed dose (if applicable). There's also a space for bedtime and snack test readings. Finally, a comments area is available for notes on special circumstances that may have affected your blood sugar that day, such as exercise, specific foods, and illness. Logbooks come in many configurations, and may also include space for checking off oral medication doses, a record of food intake for each meal, and detailed information on daily exercise. Try out a few formats until you find one that works well for you.

Daily Diabetes Log

Week of: _____

Day	Breakfast		Lunch		Dinner		Bedtime		Other/Snack		Comments
	Pre / Post	Carbs / Insulin	Pre / Post	Carbs / Insulin	Pre / Post	Carbs / Insulin	Pre / Post	Carbs / Insulin	Pre / Post	Carbs / Insulin	Diet, exercise, ketones, illness, stress
Mon		/		/		/		/		/	
Tue		/		/		/		/		/	
Wed		/		/		/		/		/	
Thu		/		/		/		/		/	
Fri		/		/		/		/		/	
Sat		/		/		/		/		/	
Sun		/		/		/		/		/	
Avg.											

Always record your blood sugar readings in a logbook, along with medication, food intake, and other important treatment notes.

Companion Software and Apps

An increasing number of meter manufacturers are putting out monitors with companion software that analyzes glucose readings for both patients and their doctors. This software can be an excellent tool for charting long-term progress of glucose control, especially if it has the ability to generate printable reports and charts, and to graph trends. Often, a special cable is required for connecting the meter to your computer and downloading data.

You can also purchase third-party software to track and analyze your blood glucose readings, or subscribe to one of the many online logging programs available on the Internet. Some programs will also record related information like blood pressure readings, cholesterol levels, carbohydrate intake, and more.

Another new trend is the advent of blood sugar tracking apps that can be used on smartphones and mobile devices. These apps have the added advantage of being integrated into a device that users are already familiar with and always carry with them. They can also easily save and analyze data.

Ways to Reduce the "Ouch" Factor

One of the biggest deterrents to frequent testing is the pain and soreness caused by finger sticks. Recently, the most significant and widely available innovation to help solve that problem is the alternative site monitor, which allows the patient to replace finger sticks with blood drawn in less sensitive areas of the body such as the forearm and thigh.

These meters may require smaller blood samples than traditional models, but as previously discussed, the readings they give may not be as accurate as those from fingertip readings

Continuous Glucose Monitoring Systems

As the name implies, a continuous glucose monitoring (CGM) system is a device that takes a glucose reading every few minutes over a period of days. By compiling glucose readings, calculating averages, and identifying trends, it can help the wearer gain valuable ongoing insight into diabetes control.

The device also has lower and upper limit alarms that can warn the user of hypoglycemia or hyperglycemia. A CGM system is designed to supplement—and not to replace—regular self-monitoring of blood glucose. These devices require regular calibration with finger stick testing.

As of mid-2012, two FDA-approved stand-alone CGM products—the DexCom Seven Plus (DexCom) and the Guardian Real-Time (Medtronic Diabetes) are available on the U.S. market. A third FDA-approved CGM, the MiniMed Paradigm Real-Time Revel (Medtronic Diabetes), is actually an insulin pump with an integrated CGM. The Guardian Real-Time measures glucose levels every five minutes for up to three days (when the sensor must be replaced).

All continuous glucose monotoring systems consist of a sensor, which is inserted just under the skin; a transmitter that connects to the sensor; and a control module that stores and displays the blood glucose data. The sensor reads glucose levels in interstitial fluid, not in blood. Consequently, the values lag approximately ten to fifteen minutes behind blood glucose levels. The testing data is sent wirelessly through the transmitter to the control module. The unit displays real-time glucose readings, alarms for preset blood sugar highs or lows, and graphs of blood glucose trends.

ALERT

Don't rely on a CGM unit to detect a blood sugar low. CGM measures glucose in interstitial fluid and the values it displays lag ten to fifteen minutes behind blood glucose values. Always use a finger stick test to detect and monitor treatment of a low.

The DexCom Seven Plus (DexCom) is a CGM system that can be used continually for seven days before reinsertion of a new sensor is required. Like the Guardian Real-Time (Medtronics Diabetes), it consists of a sensor worn just under the skin; a wireless transmitter; and a unit for receiving, analyzing, and displaying the results. It also displays current readings, trend graphs, and alarms. Both the Seven Plus and the Guardian require calibration every twelve hours.

CHAPTER 8

Type 2 Medications

If you have type 2 diabetes, you may not need to rely on insulin injections, but there may be times, however, when despite all your best efforts and commitment to diet and regular exercise, your blood glucose levels just won't stay down. According to the Centers for Disease Control (CDC), only an estimated 16 percent of American adults treat their type 2 diabetes with diet and exercise alone. The next line of defense is medication.

The Basics

If you're having trouble managing your type 2 diabetes with diet and exercise alone, your doctor may prescribe medication to improve your blood glucose control. While some people with type 2 diabetes may require insulin treatment at some point, oral medications are typically given an adequate trial first. However, in some cases, insulin may be prescribed earlier. Sometimes insulin therapy will be combined with an oral medication to improve its effectiveness. There are also several new noninsulin injectable medications on the market, described later in this chapter, that may be recommended by your doctor.

ALERT

Make sure that your doctor is aware of all other medications—prescription, over-the-counter, or herbal—that you are taking. The therapeutic action of your diabetes drug may be either increased or reduced when taken along with certain substances and medicines.

There are eight classes of oral medications for type 2 diabetes: sulfonylureas, biguanides, thiazolidinediones (also called TZDs or glitizones), alpha-glucosidase inhibitors, meglitinides, DPP-4 inhibitors, centrally acting dopamine agonists, and bile acid sequestrants. Doctors also prescribe combination drugs, which combine medications across two classes of drugs. Diabetes drugs that are currently on the U.S. market work in one of several ways:

- By inhibiting glucose production by the liver (biguanides, DPP-4 inhibitors)
- By increasing insulin sensitivity (TZDs)
- By stimulating insulin production (DPP-4 inhibitors, meglitinides, sulfonylureas)
- By blocking or slowing the digestion of carbohydrates (alpha-glucosidase inhibitors)
- By increasing activity in the dopamine receptors of the brain where neuroendocrine functions are controlled (centrally acting dopamine agonists)
- Through a combination of two or more of the actions described (combination drugs)

The mechanism by which some diabetes drugs lower blood glucose is not yet completely understood. Welchol (colesevelam hydrochloride), for example, is a drug that was first approved for high cholesterol. But researchers discovered that the drug was also effective in lowering the A1C, or long-term blood sugar measurement, of people with diabetes. While the underlying reason for this helpful side effect is not known, the drug has since been approved for diabetes treatment as well.

A Smooth Start

When you start on a new medication, log both the amount and timing of the dosage in your blood sugar logbook. This will give you and your health care provider a good idea of the impact the drug is having, and will allow her to make any necessary adjustments. You should note the side effects, if any, you have from the drug as well. Some side effects will often wane and even disappear completely as your body becomes accustomed to the medication. In some cases, however, a dosage or medication change may eventually be required.

Your doctor should explain both the amount and frequency of your dose and any specific instructions about when to take it. However, it's also a good idea to read the drug labeling and directions for use that your pharmacist provides to ensure that you're taking your medication at the appropriate time and dosage. If the printed instructions seem to vary from what you have been told, call your physician immediately for instructions.

ESSENTIAL

If your prescription is pricey, ask if a generic version is available. Drug manufacturers also provide a number of patient assistance programs for people who can't afford their diabetes medications.

Practical Matters

Medication won't work if you forget to take it, so put your meds in a place where they are in sight and on your mind. If you take several prescription drugs, a medication organizer may be a good investment for you. There are many on the market, ranging from simple plastic caddies to more elaborate electronic systems. A watch with an audible alarm can also help keep you on track. Some people find it convenient to keep their medication with their blood glucose testing supplies. If you're prescribed a drug that must be taken with meals, keep it on the kitchen table or counter. You should also carry several pills in your purse, car, or another "always with you" spot for meals on the road. Make sure you rotate your extras weekly so they don't expire.

Keeping meds within arm's reach can be hazardous in households with small children. Try keeping an empty pill bottle on the table as your reminder, and stow the full bottle in a childproof cabinet.

Finally, always avoid storing your medications in heat, humidity, or direct sunlight, as temperature extremes can cause some drugs to lose their potency. And never take a drug that is past its expiration date.

Sulfonylureas

Sulfonylureas are the oldest class of oral diabetes medication, and were first introduced in the 1950s. Brand names of these drugs include Amaryl (glimepiride), DiaBeta (glyburide), Diabinese (chlorpropamide), Dymelor (acetohexamide), Glucotrol (glipizide), Glucotrol XL (glipizide), Glynase PresTab (glyburide), and Micronase (glyburide). The generic sulfonylureas tolbutamide and tolazamide are also available, but are prescribed infrequently.

The oldest sulfonylurea drugs—Diabinese, tolbutamide, and tolazamide —require the largest dosage sizes (with daily doses ranging from 100 to 3,000 milligrams). The newer, or second-generation, sulfonylureas are much more potent. These second-generation drugs are usually taken once daily; your doctor will tell you when and how often to take your medication. Whatever the schedule, you should always try to take your medication consistently at the same time from day to day.

How They Work

Called hypoglycemic agents, sulfonylurea drugs primarily work by causing the pancreas to release more insulin, which in turn lowers blood glucose levels. For this reason, sulfonylureas may not be effective in people with long-standing diabetes who have lost most pancreatic beta cell function. Some sulfonylureas such as Amaryl (glimepiride), and Glucotrol, also work to decrease insulin resistance by binding with insulin receptors. So in addition to increasing insulin output, these drugs allow the body to more effectively use the insulin it produces.

Possible Side Effects

The most serious potential side effect of the sulfonylurea drugs is a hypoglycemic reaction, or low blood sugar episode. The older sulfonylureas, in particular, are more likely to cause this reaction if taken in conjunction with other medications. Patients taking some of these first-generation drugs may run an increased chance of cardiovascular problems, so anyone with a history of heart problems should speak with his or her doctor about the potential risks.

Other possible side effects include, but are not limited to, the following:

- Nausea
- Rash and/or itching
- Photosensitivity (skin sensitivity to sunlight)
- Dizziness
- Drowsiness
- Headache
- Weight gain

The potential for weight gain can be a problem for overweight patients, as weight gain will work against the benefits of the drug by increasing insulin resistance. Your physician may prefer to use a different class of drugs, such as biguanides, for your treatment if you are significantly overweight. Sulfonylureas (particularly chlorpropamide) also have the potential to react with alcohol, causing nausea, vomiting, and facial flushing. If you drink, talk to your doctor about this side effect before starting your prescription.

Biguanides

The biguanide class of drugs—Glucophage (metformin), Glucophage XR (metformin hydrochloride, extended release), Glumetza, and Riomet (liquid metformin)—is one of the most widely prescribed for type 2 diabetes. Biguanides are often preferred over sulfonylureas because they don't cause hypoglycemia nor do they promote weight gain. They have also been shown to have a positive effect on blood lipid levels.

Metformin is usually taken two to three times daily with meals. The extended release version is designed for once-a-day use, usually with an evening meal. It may also be used in conjunction with a sulfonylurea drug (the combination drug Glucovance is both metformin and glyburide) or with insulin therapy.

How They Work

Metformin works by suppressing the amount of glucose your liver pumps out, and consequently reduces the amount of insulin produced by the body. This drug also increases liver, muscle, and fat sensitivity to insulin. Metformin does not promote weight gain (as some type 2 drugs do) and may improve cholesterol profiles in some patients.

Possible Side Effects

Metformin is contraindicated, or not recommended, for many people with kidney or liver problems due to the risk of lactic acidosis, a rare but potentially fatal buildup of lactic acid in the bloodstream that occurs when the kidneys do not adequately remove lactic acid. Your doctor can advise you whether the drug is appropriate for you if you have kidney or liver impairment.

Signs of lactic acidosis include weakness, fatigue, dizziness, breathing problems, and unexplained muscle and/or stomach pain. If you experience any of these symptoms while taking metformin and suspect lactic acidosis, call your doctor immediately or go to the nearest emergency care facility.

FACT

Metformin, the first line treatment for type 2 diabetes, has also shown promise as a possible therapy for cancer and cancer prevention. Possible applications include prostate, breast, and colon cancer. Researchers believe the drug may help by lowering circulating levels of insulin in the body.

Biguanides are also not recommended for use in patients with congestive heart failure. Other potential side effects of metformin include the following:

- Gastrointestinal distress (gas and diarrhea)
- Nausea
- Metallic taste in the mouth
- Depletion of vitamin B_{12} levels

Because up to 30 percent of patients who are prescribed metformin experience gastrointestinal discomfort, dosage is generally started quite low, and then slowly increased. The extended-release versions of metaformin are less likely to cause gastrointestinal side effects.

ALERT

If you are undergoing any radiographic (i.e., X-ray or CT scan) procedure that involves injection of a contrast medium (dye) that contains iodine, you should stop taking metformin temporarily because of the risk of lactic acidosis. You can start taking metformin again if kidney function is normal when reassessed forty-eight hours after the injection.

Thiazolidinediones (TZDs)

Actos (pioglitazone) is the only thiazolidinedione (TZD) drug widely available in the United States. The Food and Drug Administration (FDA) has approved Actos for use with insulin, metformin, or sulfonylurea drugs. It is typically taken once daily.

A second drug, Avandia (rosiglitazone), was withdrawn from general retail pharmacy sale in late 2011 following several large-scale studies that associated the drug with an increased risk of heart attack. Avandia is now only available through a special access program administered by GlaxoSmithKline, the drug's manufacturer. The Avandia-Rosiglitazone Medicines Access Program covers Avandia and the rosiglitazone combination drugs Avandamet and Avandaryl, and is only open to those patients with type 2 diabetes who were successfully treated with these drugs previously, or who have not been able to control their blood sugar with any other medications.

How They Work

The TZD drugs, which are also called glitazones or insulin sensitizers, target the insulin receptors in muscle and fat cells to increase the level of insulin sensitivity in the body. These drugs reduce glucose production by the liver (to a small extent) and are also effective in controlling blood pressure. Some TZDs also may be helpful in lowering triglyceride levels and in increasing HDL (or "good") cholesterol.

Possible Side Effects

The use of Actos for more than a year has been associated with an increased risk of bladder cancer. People on higher doses of Actos for longer periods of time seem to be at the greatest risk for bladder cancer. Anyone with a history of bladder cancer or being treated for the condition should not take Actos.

And as previously mentioned, Avandia has been associated with an increased cardiovascular mortality risk in several large trials of type 2 patients. If you take Avandia, you should talk to your doctor about your overall risk of cardiovascular problems and whether or not the drug is right for you.

FACT

If you take birth control pills, TZD drugs can make them less effective. They can also increase fertility in women with polycystic ovary syndrome (PCOS). Women who take TZD drugs should speak with their doctor about contraceptive options.

TZD drugs have also been linked to congestive heart failure (CHF), and they are known to make pre-existing CHF worse. Patients with CHF should not take any TZD drug. If your doctor starts you on a TZD, or increases your dose, you and your doctor should watch carefully for signs of edema (swelling), sudden rapid weight gain, and dyspnea (severe shortness of breath)—all symptoms of heart failure.

If you take a TZD, you must also have regular testing of the liver enzymes ALT/AST. Liver enzyme levels should be tested before treatment starts, every two months for the first year you take the drug, and as recommended by your doctor thereafter. TZDs should be discontinued if liver enzyme levels rise more than three times the normal upper limit, and should not be started in patients who have ALT levels that are greater than 2.5 times higher than the normal upper limit.

Other side effects of TZD therapy may include the following:

- Anemia
- Weight gain
- Muscle weakness
- Headaches
- Fatigue
- Cold-like symptoms

Alpha-Glucosidase (AG) Inhibitors

The alpha-glucosidase (AG) inhibitor class of type 2 drugs consists of Glyset (miglitol) and Precose (acarbose). Also called starch blockers, these medications must be taken at each meal with the first bite of food in order to be effective. AG inhibitors may be prescribed along with a sulfonylurea drug, metformin, or insulin for some patients.

ALERT

If a blood sugar low occurs when Glyset or Precose is taken in conjunction with a sulfonylurea or insulin, it should be treated with glucose gel or tablets. AG inhibitors slow the digestion of sucrose, so things like table sugar and sucrose-containing foods are not good choices as hypoglycemic treatments.

How They Work

Glyset and Precose work by slowing digestion. More specifically, they block the enzymes that are responsible for the breakdown of carbohydrates in the intestine, so blood glucose rise is slower and steadier. They may be prescribed for you if you have a hard time keeping your postprandial (after-meal) blood glucose levels under control. AG inhibitors may be a preferred therapy in overweight patients, since they do not promote weight gain like the sulfonylureas and TZDs do.

Possible Side Effects

Because of the way they work, the AG inhibitors' side effects are primarily gastrointestinal, and include bloating, diarrhea, gas, and cramping. However, like metformin, these uncomfortable side effects can be greatly reduced by starting with a small dose and gradually increasing it. People with serious gastrointestinal disorders, including intestinal disease or obstructions, inflammatory bowel disease, and colonic ulceration, should not take AG inhibitors.

Meglitinides

Prandin (repaglinide) and Starlix (nateglinide) are currently the only FDA-approved meglitinide class drugs in the United States. Like AG inhibitors, they are taken at mealtimes (usually about fifteen minutes before eating) to prevent a postprandial (after-meal) blood sugar rise. People who tend to test high after meals may benefit from treatment with meglitinide drugs.

Prandin is also FDA-approved for use with the insulin sensitizers Actos (pioglitazone) and Avandia (rosiglitazone) and for use with metformin. Starlix is cleared for use with metformin.

How They Work

Meglitinides are short-acting oral hypoglycemic agents that bind to and stimulate the insulin-producing beta cells of the pancreas. Taken before a meal, these drugs can boost what is known as first-phase insulin release—the production of insulin that is a response to the initial boost of carb-generated blood glucose after a meal. Both Prandin and Starlix can be taken anytime from thirty minutes prior to a meal to right before the meal.

Possible Side Effects

Hypoglycemia can occur as a side effect of the meglitinide drugs. Symptoms of a low blood glucose episode include sweating, shakiness, dizziness, increased appetite, disorientation, heart palpitations, nausea, fatigue, and weakness. Hypoglycemia should be treated immediately with a fast-acting carbohydrate. Patients new to type 2 medications may also experience weight gain with meglitinides. The most commonly reported side effects that occur with meglitinide drugs are the following:

- Cold and flu symptoms
- Headache
- Diarrhea and other gastrointestinal complaints
- Joint and back pain

If you take a meglitinide drug, you should monitor your blood sugar levels either one or two hours after eating to ensure your medication is working properly. If blood sugar readings still seem too high, talk to your doctor about adjusting your dose.

QUESTION

If I skip a meal, should I still take my meds?
Try not to skip meals, as it's hard on blood sugar control. That said, it depends on the type of medication you take and when you take it. If you take an AG inhibitor or a meglitinide, you should skip the dose and take the next one with your next meal. As always, talk to your doctor about your specific situation.

Dipeptidyl Peptidase-4 (DPP-4) Inhibitors

The first DPP-4 inhibitor, Januvia (sitagliptin, by Merck), was approved in 2006 for use in type 2 adults. Onglyza (saxagliptin, by Bristol-Myers Squibb and AstraZeneca) followed in 2009, and Tradjenta (linagliptin, Boehringer Ingelheim and Eli Lilly) received FDA approval in 2011.

All the DPP-4 inhibitors are taken once daily. This class of drug helps to stimulate insulin production while suppressing glucagon production by the pancreas, thereby decreasing the amount of glucose in the body.

These drugs generally do not cause weight gain and are not associated with hypoglycemia when used alone. And unlike some other oral medications, they have a very low incidence of gastrointestinal side effects (e.g., nausea, vomiting, diarrhea). This makes DPP-4 inhibitors a good choice for many people with type 2 diabetes.

How They Work

Dipeptidyl peptidase-4 (DPP-4) is a naturally occurring enzyme that breaks down incretins, which are hormones generated during the digestive process. Incretins bind to beta cell receptors on the pancreas, stimulating the release of insulin. The incretin known as glucagon-like peptide-1 (or GLP-1) also helps to suppress the production of glucagon by the pancreas (and subsequent glucose release by the liver). But after GLP-1 is released by the gut, it only lasts about two minutes in the human body before it is broken down by DPP-4. Drugs in the DPP-4 inhibitor class block the action of the DPP-4 enzyme, which helps these important incretins regulate blood glucose levels by increasing insulin production and lowering glucagon output.

Side Effects

Headache, sore throat, muscle pain, and minor respiratory problems are the most commonly reported side effects of all of the DPP-4 drugs. Respiratory problems range from nasopharyngitis (stuffy or runny nose) to upper respiratory tract infection.

DPP-4 inhibitor use has also been linked to an increased risk of pancreatitis. Anyone with a history of pancreatitis, gallstones, or high triglyceride levels should let their doctor know, as DPP-4 inhibitors may not be a good choice for them.

Because DPP-4 is a relatively new drug class, further long-term research and follow-up studies are needed to determine the full range of potential side effects and risks associated with these drugs.

Centrally-Acting Agonist Inhibitors

Cycloset (bromocriptine mesylate, by Santarus) is the first in a new class of drugs that works by influencing brain activity. The drug is taken once a day with food—first thing in the morning when dopamine in the brain is at its lowest level—and lowers blood sugar levels without increasing insulin production by the body. The drug is often prescribed with other diabetes medicines (metformin, sulfonylureas, or TZDs) to manage postprandial (after meal) blood sugar spikes.

How They Work

Although Cycloset has undergone clinical trials and is FDA approved, researchers still don't completely understand what makes the drug effective in lowering blood sugar levels. They do know that the drug increases dopamine activity in the brain, which is thought to be the mechanism by which it works. People with type 2 diabetes appear to have lower levels of dopamine activity in the morning, and the theory is that these low levels are directly related to their body's ability to control blood sugar.

Side Effects

The most common side effects of Cycloset are low blood sugar, nausea, dizziness, fatigue, and headaches. The drug can also lower blood pressure levels, so if you are taking medicines to treat hypertension, your doctor should monitor you carefully in case you need to make adjustments to your treatment. If you have hypotension (or low blood pressure) or a history of syncopal migraines, Cycloset may not be a good choice for you. It can also cause sleepiness after you take your drug dose, so do not drive or operate heavy machinery immediately after taking Cycloset.

If you take other medicines and Cycloset is prescribed to you, make sure your doctor knows what they are. Cycloset can interact with certain drugs.

Bile Acid Sequesterants

Bile acid sequesterants are drugs that work in the gastrointestinal tract to lower cholesterol levels. Welchol (cosevelam) is the only current drug in this class approved for the treatment of type 2 diabetes. The medication was first introduced in the year 2000 as a therapy to lower LDL (bad) cholesterol levels, and it is still prescribed for that purpose. After studies showed its effectiveness in lowering A1C levels, the FDA also cleared it for use as an adjunct (or additive) therapy for type 2 in 2008. Welchol is typically prescribed along with metformin and can be an effective treatment choice for people who need to lower their LDL levels along with their A1C.

How They Work

Researchers aren't sure exactly what makes bile acid sequesterants effective in lowering blood sugar levels. Some have hypothesized that the drugs cause the liver to reduce glucose production. It has also been suggested that they may increase secretion of incretin hormones that lower blood sugar levels.

The reason bile acid sequesterants are effective in lowering LDL levels is because they increase the amount of bile acids excreted from the body and decrease those acids returning to the liver. The liver reacts to the deficit by synthesizing more bile acids from cholesterol, which reduces levels of cholesterol in the blood.

Side Effects

The most common side effects of Welchol are gastrointestinal, specifically constipation and upset stomach. People with a history of bowel obstructions should not take the drug, and anyone with diabetic gastroparesis should be followed closely when taking Welchol. Welchol can increase triglyceride levels, particularly in people already taking sulfonylurea drugs or insulin—so anyone with high triglycerides (>300) should use Welchol with caution.

Other Injectables

Exenatide (Byetta; Bydureon), liraglutide (Victoza), and pramlintide (Symlin) are injectable drugs. Byetta and Victoza are part of a class of drugs known as *incretin mimetics* that work by "mimicking" the action of hormones called incretins, which are key in regulating blood glucose levels. Symlin is a synthetic version of amylin, a neuroendocrine hormone (i.e., hormones that regulate interactions between the endocrine and nervous systems) that also plays a major role in blood glucose regulation.

Byetta is approved for use either by itself or in combination with metformin, a sulfonylurea, a TZD, or Lantus (insulin glargine). It is usually prescribed when a patient is unable to achieve control with oral medications or Lantus alone.

Byetta is not a substitute for insulin, and type 2 diabetes patients who are already on insulin should not stop taking insulin to try Byetta. The long-acting insulin Lantus is currently the only insulin approved for use with Byetta; and Byetta should not be taken with short or rapid acting insulins.

Byetta injections are taken twice daily up to an hour before a major meal. Most people prefer to take it before breakfast and dinner, but any two mealtimes are fine as long as there are six hours between them. An extended-release formulation of the drug Byetta, called Bydureon, was approved by the FDA in January 2012. Bydureon only requires a once weekly injection.

Victoza is injected once a day, either with or without food. The drug may be taken alone or in combination with metformin, sulfonyurea, or TZD drugs. Injectable medications such as incretin mimetics and Symlin should be injected at separate sites from other injectable medication (such as insulin). These medications may interfere with each other, resulting in decreased effectiveness of both. Victoza is also approved for use with long-lasting basal insulin.

ALERT

If you skip a meal, you should also skip your Byetta or Symlin injection. And if you forget to take the injection before eating, do not take it after the meal. Instead, wait until your next scheduled mealtime dose.

Symlin is used as an adjunct (or companion) treatment to insulin. It is available in vials and pens, and is injected right before any major meal (i.e., at least 30 grams of carbs and/or 250 calories). While both rapid-acting insulin and Symlin may be injected prior to a meal, insulin and Symlin should never be administered in the same syringe, as mixing these drugs alters the chemical composition of Symlin. If your doctor starts you on Symlin, he will reduce your premeal insulin dose by up to 50 percent, depending on the type of insulin you use.

How They Work

Byetta, Victoza, and Symlin have some similar features. First, they slow the rate of stomach emptying and send "all full" signals to the brain that promote feelings of satiety. They also help control blood sugar levels by suppressing glucagon production by the liver. Byetta and Victoza have an additional trick up their sleeve. These drugs also stimulate insulin production in the pancreas. This only happens when elevated blood glucose is detected, so they do not cause low blood sugars.

Byetta and Victoza mimic the action of the incretin GLP-1, which is secreted by the intestines in response to food digestion. Incretins help to stimulate insulin production in the pancreas, and certain types of incretins also work to suppress glucagon production in the pancreas. These drugs may also restore what is known as first phase insulin response—high levels of insulin secretion that occur in the first ten minutes after glucose is detected.

Side Effects

Byetta, Victoza, and Symlin are neither designed nor FDA-approved as weight-loss drugs, but weight loss is one of the side effects of these medications. In clinical trials, people on Byetta lost an average of five pounds in thirty weeks. Nausea is one of the most reported side effects of all three drugs, which may explain why weight loss occurs.

Because these drugs slow gastric emptying, they should not be used by people with gastroparesis. They can also slow the body's absorption of other drugs and consequently affect their therapeutic action. Make sure your health care team is aware if you start treatment on any of these medications.

Byetta is not recommended for use in patients with severe renal impairment or end-stage renal disease. There have also been postmarket reports (patient reports that occur after a drug has been FDA approved) of pancreatitis in some Byetta users. Severe abdominal pain, sometimes with vomiting, is the main symptom of pancreatitis; if you experience this while on Byetta, let your doctor know immediately.

Patients taking Victoza should heed the same warnings. This drug was associated with some cases of pancreatitis during clinical trials, and it is not clear yet if Victoza increases the risk of this condition. Victoza was also associated with the development of thyroid tumors in animal studies, and the

FDA has required the manufacturer to monitor thyroid cancer among Victoza users in order to further study this risk. Anyone with medullary thyroid cancer, or a family history of the condition, is advised not to take Victoza.

People who take Symlin are at higher risk of hypoglycemia, in part because the medication is used in conjunction with insulin. Your doctor may recommend that when you first start on Symlin, or when you adjust doses, you refrain from driving or operating heavy machinery up to three hours after taking a Symlin injection. You should also test frequently during this time. Insulin doses often have to be adjusted after initiation of Symlin therapy, so testing and logging results is particularly important during this time.

Combination Drugs

Drugs that combine two classes of medications are called combination drugs. Combination drugs available in the United States as of mid-2012 included Actoplus Met (pioglitizone and metformin), Duetact (pioglitizone and glimepiride), Glucovance (glyburide and metformin), Janumet (sitagliptin and metformin),Janumet XR (sitaglipitm and metaformin XR), Jentadueto (linagliptin and metformin), Juvisync (sitagliptin and simvastatin), Kombiglyze XR (saxagliptin and metformin XR), Metaglip (glipizide and metformin), and PrandiMet (repaglinide and metformin). Avandamet (rosiglitazone and metformin) and Avandaryl (rosiglitazone and glimepiride) are available only to certain eligible patients through the Avandia-Rosiglitazone Medicines Access Program. See the information on TZD drugs and Avandia earlier in this chapter.

Several studies have shown that some diabetes drugs may have the potential to delay or prevent type 2 diabetes. The Diabetes Prevention Program (DPP) shows that metformin reduces the risk of type 2 diabetes by 31 percent and the STOP-NIDDM trial shows that acarbose reduces the risk by 32 percent.

Metformin is the common ingredient in most of these drugs because it safely suppresses glucose production in the liver without the risk of hypoglycemia. Metformin also doesn't promote weight gain, and it improves lipid profiles in some patients. The same risks and contraindications that apply to these drugs separately are also applicable to their combination formulation. However, even if you are familiar with one component of a combination drug (i.e., metformin), you should always thoroughly read the drug's directions for use before taking it to be aware of any unknown side effects or warnings.

No Magic Pill

Prescription drugs are never a substitute for appropriate diet and exercise in the treatment of type 2 diabetes, and ignoring these other two fundamentals of diabetes management is a recipe for disaster. If and when you start medication, stay on track with your diet and exercise program. You need all three parts of this equation to manage your diabetes effectively.

On the other hand, sometimes people with type 2 diabetes hesitate to agree to drugs because they feel like they have failed if they can't achieve blood sugar control with diet and exercise alone. Remember that medication is not a crutch but rather just another tool for getting your blood glucose levels under control, which is your main objective in managing your diabetes. You need to take advantage of every tool at your disposal to build a solid and effective treatment program.

CHAPTER 9

All about Insulin

Many type 2 diabetes patients end up needing insulin to control their blood sugar. As people age, insulin resistance increases and the ability of the pancreas to produce sufficient insulin drops, making insulin treatment more likely for type 2 patients. This is part of the natural progress of diabetes. Even so, many patients still avoid insulin due to unfounded fears and misperceptions about the drug. It's important to recognize insulin for what it is—a powerful tool for normalizing blood sugar levels and stopping diabetes complications.

Insulin Is Not a Sign of Failure

Insulin can be one of the most effective tools in controlling type 2 diabetes. Yet despite the proven benefits, many people fear and avoid it, damaging their health in the process. It's clear from large scale, long-term studies like the United Kingdom Prospective Diabetes Study (UKPDS) that A1C levels above 7 percent can greatly increase the incidence of eye, kidney, and nerve vascular damage over time.

But despite all our health care providers may say about the benefits of good blood sugar control, on average, a patient with type 2 diabetes who is not in control will spend five years with their A1C over 8 percent and ten years with it over 7 percent before they will agree to go on insulin therapy. Why the disconnect? Fear and misinformation are at the root of the problem for most patients who refuse insulin. Often referred to as "psychological insulin resistance," the mental barriers people face when confronted with the idea of transitioning to insulin therapy can feel significant. Barriers include the following:

- **Feelings of failure.** Insulin is often perceived as a punishment for bad diabetes control behavior. People often feel that they have "failed" at controlling their diabetes, and had they just exercised more, eaten less, or tried different drugs, they may not be facing the insulin choice. The truth is that in type 2 diabetes, your body's ability to produce insulin will diminish over time, and a transition to insulin only reflects this natural progression.
- **Fear of deteriorating health.** Some people feel that a move to insulin is the beginning of the end, and marks a worsening of the disease. In fact, insulin may be the best choice for improving your diabetes health because it better controls blood sugar levels.
- **Fear of blood sugar lows.** While it is true that insulin can cause hypoglycemia, or blood sugar lows, with proper education and precautions these are easily avoided. Knowing how to quickly and effectively treat a "hypo" is the best defense against living in fear of low blood sugar episodes.
- **Fear of weight gain.** Yes, insulin can cause weight gain. No, this is not an inevitable outcome, especially for people who pay attention to the other two foundations of good diabetes care—eating right and getting regular exercise.

- **Fear of injections.** Of all the fears of insulin, this is probably the one with the least basis in reality. Today's insulin needles are so small and fine that the needle stick is barely noticeable. In fact, most people say that a lancet stick for blood sugar testing causes more discomfort than an insulin syringe or pen stick. As part of the insulin teaching process, many health care providers will actually inject themselves, using saline, to show their patients how easy and pain-free the process is.
- **Embarrassment.** Many people still fear what they consider the social stigma of injecting insulin in public. But with today's insulin pens, where taking insulin is as easy as dialing up a dose and pushing a button, insulin can be discreetly and quickly injected with no muss or fuss.
- **Inconvenience.** Insulin therapy may mean you have a little more gear to carry around. But again, with the simplicity of insulin pens, and especially with once or twice daily long-acting insulin doses, it's a small price to pay for better diabetes health.

FACT

Inaccuracies and missed doses are not uncommon among people with type 2 on insulin. The GAPP2 (Global Attitude of Patients and Physicians) study, a survey of type 2 patients in six countries, found that 22 percent had missed a basal insulin dose and 24 percent had mistimed their dose in the previous thirty days.

How Does Insulin Work?

Injected insulin mimics the action of the hormone normally produced by the body. Once insulin is injected under the skin and into the subcutaneous (below the skin) fat layer, it starts stimulating glucose uptake by both skeletal muscle and fat cells, while at the same time signaling the liver to slow or stop glucose production. So in effect, it closes one door (the liver) while opening another (the body cells).

The first insulin, isolated in 1922 by Canadians Sir Frederick Banting and Charles Best (with help from fellow researchers J. J. R. Macleod and J. B. Collip), was extracted from the pancreas of a cow. The first few decades of insulin therapy used both bovine (cow) and porcine (pig) derived insulin.

Today's insulins are created in the laboratory, cultured from bacteria and yeast with a technology known as recombinant DNA.

FACT

Before the discovery of insulin in the 1920s, the only way to treat diabetes was through a near-starvation diet, and patients consequently did not have a very long life span. Today, electronically programmed pumps can deliver precise doses of the life-saving hormone, and new noninvasive forms of delivering insulin are on the horizon.

Insulin Types and Quantities

Insulin comes in several different strengths and actions. Long-acting (basal) insulin products such as insulin glargine (Lantus) and detemir (Levemir) are designed to provide up to twenty-four-hour "peakless" coverage. These are frequently prescribed for people with type 2 diabetes starting on insulin therapy. An even longer-acting basal insulin, degludec, is designed to last thirty-six hours, but is not yet approved in the United States (as of mid-2012).

Sometimes mealtime insulin will be recommended for type 2 patients who are having difficulty keeping their postprandial (or after meal) blood sugar levels under control. Rapid-acting insulin such as Humalog, NovoLog, or Apidra is injected before a meal and starts working in fewer than fifteen minutes. Its peak of action (when it is working the hardest) is between thirty to ninety minutes after injection, about the time when blood sugar levels would be at their height after a meal.

Regular insulin starts working thirty to sixty minutes after injection and peaks a bit later than rapid-acting insulin. NPH insulins are longer lasting and have a slower onset and peak action. They are often used in combination with regular insulins. Insulin mixes can also be used to "cover" a meal; and combine longer-lasting NPH insulin with regular acting insulin in different amounts.

It's important to note that onset, peak, and duration vary from person to person, and can be influenced by other health conditions a person may have, as well as weight. You and your doctor will choose an appropriate insulin or mix of insulin products based on your particular needs and blood sugar patterns.

ESSENTIAL

"Insulin onset" is how long it takes the insulin to start affecting blood sugar levels. "Insulin peak" is the time frame that it takes for the insulin to reach its maximum efficacy. And the "insulin duration" is the overall length of time insulin works to lower blood sugar levels.

The insulin mixes (i.e., 75/25, 70/30, 50/50) are convenient, commonly prescribed insulin combinations. These mixes eliminate your chances of making an error when trying to draw up two different insulin types. They are also a boon to those people who may have vision or dexterity problems or find mixing insulins difficult for other reasons.

Insulin Dosage

Your insulin dose will depend on the type and action of your insulin. Your doctor will tell you exactly what kind and how much insulin to inject, and when you should be taking it. If you take a long-acting insulin like Lantus or Levemir, you will be injecting once or twice daily.

However, if you take a mealtime insulin, your doctor or diabetes educator will teach you how to determine the amount of regular or rapid-acting insulin you need based on how many carbohydrates you are going to eat. This is called "covering carbohydrates" and you'll have to do a little bit of math to determine your dose.

This kind of premeal insulin dosing is based on something called the insulin-to-carbohydrate ratio. Everyone has their own unique ratio, but the rule of thumb is that each unit of regular insulin covers about 15 grams of carbs (the insulin-to-carbohydrate ratio). For every 50 mg/dl blood sugar is above the target range, an additional unit of insulin should be added (the blood sugar-to-insulin ratio). So if you were planning on eating a dinner that has 90 carbs and your blood sugar was 100 mg/dl over target, 8 units of insulin would be necessary (6 to cover the carbs and 2 for the blood sugar). Remember, this is a general guideline only; the insulin-to-carb ratio is different for everyone, as is the insulin-to-blood sugar ratio, and you should work with your diabetes health care provider to track your glucose levels and determine what ratios are right for you.

Selecting the Insulin Delivery Device

Insulin must be injected into your body's subcutaneous layer of fat. As of mid-2012, the available devices for administering insulin were syringes, insulin pens, ports, pumps, and air-propelled "jet" injection devices. The type of delivery device you choose will depend on your insulin prescription, budget, insurance coverage, and comfort level.

Choosing a Syringe

Syringes are probably the least expensive option for injecting insulin. They are readily available at virtually any pharmacy and are easy to operate. If your insulin regimen requires mixing two types of insulin that aren't commonly available in a premixed pen, a syringe is your only choice.

Syringes come in a variety of sizes and needle gauges, from 30 to 100 units ($1/33$ of a cc to 1 cc), with needles ranging in length from 4–12 mm. Some come with half-unit markings. When you're shopping for syringes, make sure you choose a type with markings that are easy for you to read and that accommodate your regular dosage.

▼ INSULINS BY TYPE, ONSET, PEAK, AND DURATION

Type	Onset	Peak	Duration
Rapid Acting			
Humalog (lispro)	<15 min.	30–90 min.	<5 hours
NovoLog (aspart)	5–20 min.	40–50 min.	3–5 hours
Apidra (glulisine)	5–15 min.	30–90 min.	<5 hours
Regular (R)			
Humulin R*	30–60 min.	3 hours	8 hours
Novolin R	30 min.	2.5–5.0 hours	8 hours
NPH			
Humulin N*	2–4 hours	4–10 hours	up to 24 hours
Novolin N	90 min.	4–12 hours	up to 24 hours
Premixed			
Humalog 75/25	15 min.	1–6.5 hours	up to 22 hours
Humalog 50/50	15 min.	1–5 hours	up to 24 hours
Humulin 70/30*	15–30 min.	1.5–16 hours	up to 24 hours

Type	Onset	Peak	Duration
Novolin 70/30	30 min.	2–12 hours	up to 24 hours
NovoLog Mix 70/30	15 min.	1–4 hours	up to 24 hours
Basal			
Lantus (glargine)	2–4 hours	minimal	up to 24 hours
Levemir (detemir)	1–4 hours	minimal	up to 24 hours

Compiled from Eli Lilly and Company, Novo Nordisk A/S, and Sanofi-Aventis U.S. product information. These are general guidelines only. A number of factors can affect insulin action, including dosage, the injection site, time of day, and exercise.

*Humulin is also sold as ReliOn at Walmart in the United States.

Insulin Pens

Pens cost more than syringes, but they have the benefit of eliminating your need to draw insulin from the vial. Instead, a pen uses a premeasured insulin cartridge, which usually contains 300 units of insulin. Pens are either disposable (one-use) models or reusable models. Reusable pens allow you to insert and dispose of insulin cartridges, which you buy separately. Both types require the use of disposable pen needles, also purchased separately.

An insulin pen resembles just that, a pen. You simply uncap it to reveal the pen needle, and then "dial up" your dose by turning the barrel until the correct number of units is displayed. After priming, you place the pen against the injection site and press a button to administer the insulin.

ALERT

Overseas, insulin dilutions and measurements are a little different, with U-40 being the standard instead of U-100. Syringes are also marked in these units. If you're traveling abroad, be aware of this important difference and bring along plenty of supplies.

Today's insulin pens are fairly discreet, and some models are designed to resemble a regular writing pen. Some newer pen models feature a display and memory module that allows you to "remember" the time of your last injection and amount of insulin you took.

Other Injection Devices

Jet injection devices use air pressure to force insulin through the skin without actually puncturing it. They are considerably more expensive than both pens and syringes, are not widely used, and can require more training to use effectively. The air pressure must be adjusted to propel the insulin strongly enough to penetrate the skin but lightly enough not to bruise. Finding a balance can take a little practice.

FACT

People who have problems with daily injections may benefit from a device called the I-port (by Patton Medical), a medication delivery system that is inserted into the skin. After the initial insertion, the port can be left in place for up to three days, and features a flexible cannula that you can inject insulin into without penetrating the skin again.

For those people who are afraid of needles, a jet injector may be a good choice. However, at a cost of several hundred dollars, they require a significant initial investment (although eventually they will pay for themselves). Some people find them bulky to carry conveniently, as they are bigger than both syringes and pens.

In 2011, a subcutaneous insulin delivery device called the V-Go (Valeritas) was approved by the FDA for use in type 2 patients taking Humalog or Novo-Log rapid acting insulin. V-Go adheres to the skin with adhesive, and similar to an insulin pump, the device disperses a basal dose (a continuous small amount of insulin throughout the day) and allows the user to administer bigger "bolus" doses with meals to cover blood sugar spikes. But unlike a pump, it has no electronic parts and is removed and replaced every twenty-four hours.

The V-Go is about the size of a deck of cards. It must be filled with insulin manually before it is applied to the body, and can be worn anywhere you might give yourself an injection (e.g., the abdomen). A button press triggers the release of a small needle into the subcutaneous tissue and starts the flow of insulin. A separate "bolus" button allows the user to administer extra units of insulin with meals.

Finally, there is the insulin pump, a sophisticated electronic device that mimics the action of the human pancreas. The pump delivers basal and bolus doses of insulin as programmed by the user. While pumps are most commonly used by people with type 1 diabetes, they are a treatment option for some people with type 2, especially for those who have difficulty managing their blood sugar by other means. The pump is covered in detail later in this chapter.

Injecting Insulin

Once you have your delivery device selected, your prescription filled, and your resolve set, you're ready to give yourself a shot. Before you start, wash your hands thoroughly and examine the bottle of insulin. If you are injecting a clear insulin like lispro, you should look for crystals, cloudiness, or debris. If you find any of these, dispose of the bottle. For users of cloudy, long-acting insulins like NPH, you will have to mix the insulin gently in the vial by rolling it back and forth between your hands about twenty times. When the color appears even, the insulin is mixed. Never shake the bottle, as this can damage the insulin.

QUESTION

What size of syringe or pen needle should I buy? There seems to be a lot of choices!
Just like testing lancets, insulin needles are available in different gauges and lengths. In general, the higher the gauge, the sharper and narrower the needle, and the less painful the stick (although skin sensitivity and injection site play a part). Needle length varies from 4mm to 12mm. Longer needles are recommended for heavier patients to prevent insulin leakage; short needles are a better choice for leaner patients who may hit muscle when injecting with longer needles.

You will also need three alcohol swabs, a syringe (or another device for injecting insulin), and a sharps disposal container.

Drawing Up the Insulin

If you don't use syringes, drawing up insulin will not be an issue. Still, it's always a good idea to know how to do it in case you're ever without your regular supplies and need to use a syringe. Syringes are a good "back up" that all diabetes patients should have on hand, just in case. Your diabetes educator and/or doctor will go over this procedure as well. Here are the basic steps:

1. Open the insulin vial or bottle and mark the date on the label.
2. Wipe off the top of the insulin vial with an alcohol swab.
3. Uncap both the plunger and the needle of the syringe.
4. Draw air into the syringe by pulling out the plunger until the stopper reaches the unit mark of what your insulin dose will be.
5. Push the syringe needle down through the rubber stopper in the insulin vial. Do not press down the plunger yet.
6. After the needle is all the way in, push the plunger all the way down to inject the air into the bottle.
7. Turn the syringe and bottle upside down. Make sure that the tip of the needle is still submerged in the insulin. If it isn't, pull the syringe out slightly until it is.
8. Slowly pull the syringe plunger out to draw the insulin until the stopper reaches the correct dosage mark.
9. Check for air bubbles. If there are some, push the insulin back in and redraw until no bubbles are visible.
10. Turn the bottle and syringe right-side up and carefully remove the syringe from the vial.

Choosing and Preparing an Injection Site

Insulin should be injected into fat to do its job properly. This makes the fatty areas of the body—the butt, abdomen, thighs, hips, and back of the upper arms—the most appropriate spots for giving injections. In general, the fatty tissue of the abdomen will absorb insulin the fastest, and is a good spot to use for mealtime insulin doses. Don't choose your bicep, calf, or any other muscular area of your body. Muscle will accelerate the speed of your insulin action, and it hurts more, too.

You can't inject yourself in the same exact spot every time. If you do, lumpy deposits of fat (lipohypertrophy) will form at the site and make injections increasingly less effective, because these deposits slow absorption of the insulin. Injection rotation doesn't require you to move from one part of the body to another; just moving over by an inch or so will do the trick. In fact, it's better to be consistent with the general area of the body you inject into (e.g., abdomen, thighs, arms) so that the absorption rate stays consistent and you can count on your insulin to start working in a certain time frame. It's good to have a method of keeping track of your rotation schedule, such as always rotating clockwise or alternating arms.

Once you have a spot picked out, clean it thoroughly. You can also wipe it with an alcohol swab to sterilize the area, although this isn't required.

Giving the Injection

Now the moment you've been waiting for—actually injecting the insulin. If you're like most people, you approach the first solo shot with trepidation, and possibly, fear. Know that you can, and will, do it. Even the most squeamish, needle-fearing patients find that a little practice has them pushing in the syringe without a second thought.

Your diabetes educator or doctor will teach you the proper method of finding a good injection site and giving yourself a shot. In fact, you may be given a syringe of saline in the office to "practice" your technique with. After you've chosen an appropriate site, follow these simple steps for giving yourself a practically painless syringe injection:

1. When you clean the area, let the alcohol dry completely before injecting to avoid a nasty sting.
2. Grab a roll of fat (or flesh) between your thumb and forefinger with your nonshooting hand. You do not want to inject into muscle, so choose appropriately.
3. Hold the syringe like a dart, paper airplane, or anything else you'd want to sail through the air. Keep your thumb off the plunger until the needle is in.
4. Assess the area where you're injecting. If it's a fairly fatty site, you can use a 90-degree angle. You can also use a 90-degree angle if you are using a very fine pen or syringe needle (such as the BD Nano). Otherwise, you may have to try up to a 45-degree angle to avoid hitting muscle or blood vessels.
5. The key to a pain-free injection is to stick the needle in completely and quickly. One caution: If you're giving insulin to a child, start a little slower. It may take some experimentation to find the speed that is least painful.
6. Depress the plunger with your thumb slowly and steadily. As you get accustomed to the "feel," adjust your speed as needed.

7. Count to five before you pull out to avoid insulin leakage. Then pull out the syringe. You're done!

QUESTION

My friend said that I could die if I injected an air bubble along with my insulin! Is that true?
Your friend was probably referring to air embolism, which can occur when air bubbles are injected into the circulatory system and block a blood vessel (this is not necessarily fatal). Since insulin is injected into the subcutaneous fat, this isn't a risk. But bubbles are bad for a different reason—they throw off your dosing.

Storing and Transporting Insulin

Hot or subzero cars, beach bags, or other extreme temperature conditions can quickly deplete insulin's potency. If you're going to be traveling or participating in a recreational activity that will expose your insulin to the elements, be sure to have an insulated case that can keep it safe.

FACT

Oral and transdermal (skin patch) insulin may someday be pain-free treatment options for U.S. diabetes patients. Oral insulin, which is delivered in a spray, has shown promise in clinical trials, because the lining of the mouth effectively absorbs insulin.

Most insulin manufacturers recommend refrigerated storage of their products. But many manufacturers state that the vial you use can be stored at room temperature (an important point, since cold insulin can be painful to inject). Always read the insulin labeling and/or manufacturer's directions for use to find out exactly what storage requirements your particular insulin has.

When Good Insulin Goes Bad

You can tell a lot about insulin by just looking at it. Always check the expiration date of your insulin before you draw it up. Then take a moment to inspect the bottle. Rapid- and short-acting insulin should be clear, while intermediate-acting insulin should look cloudy. The long-lasting insulins glargine (Lantus) and detemir (Levemir) should be clear. If your insulin has any crystals or debris in it, or looks cloudy when it should be clear, it could be either expired or spoiled. Never take a chance if it looks questionable; when in doubt, throw it out.

Of course, if you purchase insulin in prefilled pens, a visual inspection is often impossible. Make sure to check expiration dates and handle and store pens properly, and you shouldn't have any spoilage issues.

Once you open a vial of insulin, its days are numbered, no matter what the expiration date. Typically, an open vial of insulin has a thirty-day shelf life. Always read the manufacturer's directions for use to find out how long a particular type of insulin will last after it has been opened.

QUESTION

What happened to the inhaled insulin I heard about on the news?
Exubera (by Pfizer), the first FDA-approved inhaled insulin, hit the market in 2006 with much fanfare . . . and was discontinued in 2007 due to lackluster sales and poor consumer and provider acceptance. As of mid-2012, there are other inhaled insulins in development by other manufacturers, but none are yet FDA-approved.

All about Insulin Pumps

An insulin pump is a small external device, about the size of a small cell phone, that is programmed to deliver a slow, continuous infusion (basal dose) of short-acting insulin into the body. At mealtimes, the wearer programs a bolus dose to cover the carbohydrates in the food she is going to eat.

The pump itself consists of a reservoir for holding insulin, a digital display with dose and time information, and a port where the insulin leaves the unit. Most pumps are also designed with a piece of thin plastic tubing called an infusion set that hooks on to the pump and carries the insulin from the device to the body. A flexible plastic cannula or a needle is inserted just under the skin to deliver the insulin. Infusion sets must be changed every two to three days, and insertion sites must be rotated. Most people use the abdomen for insertion, although the same sites that can be used for insulin injection with a syringe can also be used for insertion.

QUESTION

What are basal and bolus doses?
A basal dose is a slow, continuous infusion of small amounts of insulin that is designed to mimic the insulin secretion of a healthy pancreas between meals. A bolus is a larger dose of insulin taken before a meal to cover the resulting rise in blood glucose levels, or a dose of insulin given to correct a high blood sugar. The bolus is computed by calculating the carbohydrates contained in the meal.

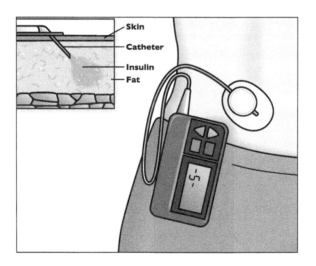

An insulin pump administers insulin through a thin catheter in the abdominal fat to help control a person's blood sugar levels.

A newer type of insulin pump, known as a patch pump, attaches directly to the skin without tubing. The first of these patch pumps, the OmniPod (from Insulet), was introduced in 2007. The OmniPod features a disposable insulin "pod" with an integrated cannula. The pod has an adhesive backing that firmly attaches to the skin around the cannula. A separate electronic device, called a personal diabetes manager (PDM), programs the insulin delivery and sends wireless signals to the pod. The PDM also doubles as a blood glucose meter and uses the results to help the user calculate insulin dosing. The insulin pods last for approximately three days; they are waterproof and can be worn in the shower. However, once attached, the pods should not be removed until replacement, so they are not as easy to "disconnect" from as a traditional pump is.

Another patch pump, the Solo (from Medingo; Roche), is FDA approved and is expected to be released for sale in the United States in late 2012. The Solo is slightly smaller than the OmniPod, and offers users the added bonus of being able to temporarily detach without having to discard the entire insulin unit. The device also allows users to bolus from a button on the insulin unit itself as well as from the handheld remote unit.

Who Pumps?

People with type 2 diabetes who are on insulin therapy may benefit from pumping if they are having trouble achieving their A1C goals with regular injection therapy. Those who suffer from nighttime lows (and accompanying morning highs) also may find that the pump helps them improve control; pumps can also be programmed to increase the basal dose as morning blood sugar levels start to rise (i.e., the dawn phenomenon).

ALERT

Be sure to read the directions for use for your particular pump thoroughly to find out its full range of capabilities. Your doctor may also have special instructions regarding pump disconnection and other issues. A professional pump trainer (often a CDE) can be invaluable in getting you off on the right foot.

An insulin pump requires a dedicated patient. It is not a "plug-and-play" solution to your diabetes management. Blood sugar levels must still be tested at least four times daily, bolus doses for meals have to be computed and programmed, and infusion sets have to be changed regularly. But people who are willing and able to put in the effort often find that the pump gives them that elusive control that injections don't.

Practical Matters

Of course, being hooked up to a pump 24/7 does bring up all sorts of daily dilemmas. The following pointers may answer the more practical questions you may be asking about pump therapy:

- **Many pumps are waterproof (to a point), or at the very least water-resistant.** So if you accidentally get them wet, you're covered. There are also a variety of special waterproof and shock-resistant cases available.
- **Infusion sets come with tubing that is several feet in length.** The extra length, which doesn't have to be used, comes in handy if you like to put your pump next to your bed at night, or even leave it out of the tub while you bathe or shower.
- **Pumps are worn to bed.** Pumps keep working even when you're sleeping. Good places to keep your pump at night are under the pillow, in a pajama pocket, or on the nightstand.
- **Pumps can be discreet.** If you don't feel comfortable wearing your pump like a beeper, there are many alternatives. Special pouches and straps to wear pumps on the body under clothing are also available.
- **Pumps can be disconnected, usually up to an hour.** If you prefer to shower, swim, or have sex without the constant companionship of your pump, you can. Always check blood sugar levels when you hook back up.

Insurance and Medicare Issues

An insulin pump is a major investment. Pumps run around $6,000 (some higher, some lower), plus the cost of infusion sets and other supplies, which can run several hundred dollars per month. The good news is that because tight control of glucose levels has been proved to reduce diabetes-related complications (as shown in the UKPDS and other trials), insurance companies are sometimes willing to cover the price of a pump early, rather than pay the price of more expensive treatment for serious complications later.

Medicare will cover insulin pumps for type 2 diabetes patients, but patients must meet strict clinical criteria to qualify. If you and your doctor think that you are a good candidate for the pump, work with him and his insurance coordinator to see if you meet Medicare guidelines.

Sharps Disposal

Insulin treatment with any form of sharps produces a lot of medical waste over time. It's important to dispose of needles and lancets properly to prevent injury to other people in your household and to anyone who comes in contact with your trash after it leaves the house. Some states and municipalities have certain requirements for medical waste disposal. When in doubt, call your public works department or trash hauler.

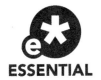

ESSENTIAL

Don't leave home without a sharps container. When you go on vacation, purchase a compact sharps disposal container before you go. Another alternative is to use a small puncture-proof case, like a pencil box or an old thermos, until you return home and can dispose of sharps properly. If you're flying, check with your airline for their policies on sharps transport.

Talk to the pharmacist where you purchase your syringes or diabetes supplies and find out if they offer a sharps bring-back or disposal program. These programs keep used sharps out of municipal landfills and incinerators where they have the potential to cause injury to workers. Ask your pharmacist if her store participates in a sharps disposal program.

If you don't have access to a sharps return program, there are many household products that come in containers that are ideal for sharps disposal. The main requirements are a puncture-resistant material and an opening that can be easily and tightly sealed. Glass is not a good choice because of the potential for breakage. Liquid laundry detergent bottles, shampoo bottles, and coffee cans (with a hole for insertion) are all good options.

Label your sharps container "Used Medical Sharps—Do Not Recycle" with a waterproof marker so everyone who comes in contact with it will handle it appropriately. Always throw sharps into your container immediately. Put one or several containers around where you tend to do your shots and testing. You can clip a needle with a specially designed safety device that is made for this purpose, but never try to cut a needle with scissors or a knife. Instead, put your sharps directly into your disposal container.

When your container is full, put the top on tightly and seal it completely with duct tape or another heavy-duty tape. Find out if your municipality has a separate procedure for medical waste and follow the guidelines they provide. If your sharps container is to be put in with the regular trash pickup, make sure it goes in the garbage can and not the recycling bin.

Insulin and Weight Gain

When blood sugar has been poorly controlled for some time, your metabolism speeds up considerably. Consequently, because the body doesn't have enough effective insulin to allow glucose into the cells, the cells go without energy and the excess glucose is diverted to the urine. At the same time, the body tries to convert fat to energy to compensate. This is why some people with extremely high blood sugars actually lose weight.

Insulin therapy normalizes metabolism and helps your body use energy from food more efficiently. Insulin allows blood sugar to enter the cells. Anything beyond what your cells need for energy will be stored as fat. As your body adjusts to these changes, weight gain is often the result. On average, people with type 2 who start on insulin therapy gain seven to eleven pounds over a three-year period. The good news is that those who are physically active tend to avoid or minimize the weight gain.

Another contributing factor to weight gain from insulin therapy is hypoglycemia. If insulin treatment hasn't been fine tuned, it's possible to experience blood sugar lows. And eating too many carbs and calories in an effort to treat these lows can result in weight gain over time. If you are having repeated episodes of hypoglycemia after starting insulin, talk to your doctor about a dose adjustment. And remember to treat lows with the 15/15 rule when they do happen. Take 15 grams of fast acting carbohydrates, like glucose tablets or gels, wait 15 minutes, and test again. If your sugar is still too low, repeat the cycle until they reach safe levels.

CHAPTER 10

Tackling Weight Loss

Over 80 percent of people with type 2 diabetes are overweight or obese. In fact, America as a nation has been packing on the pounds for the past two decades. A whopping one-third of all American adults are classified as obese, and the rate of childhood obesity is skyrocketing. Losing weight is one of the best ways to treat type 2 diabetes, but it is also possibly the most difficult.

In Control and Gaining Weight

Some of the hypoglycemic drugs prescribed for type 2 diabetes can cause weight gain in its users. Insulin-sensitizing thiazolidinediones (also called TZDs or glitazones), including Actos (pioglitazone) and Avandia (rosiglitazone), and sulfonylurea drugs fall into this category. Because TZDs can also cause edema, weight gain from their use may mean a gain in fluids rather than in fat. On the other hand, metformin can cause weight loss in some people. If you're taking one of these TZD drugs and experiencing weight gain as a side effect, your doctor may add metformin to your mix.

Combination drugs can eliminate the need for two separate prescription drugs, and so may be more convenient and less costly for some patients. Combination drugs are not an option for all type 2 patients. Talk to your doctor about whether or not they may be right for you.

A new generation of type 2 injectable drugs has also shown some capacity for encouraging weight loss. In clinical trials, the drug exenatide (Byetta; from Amylin Pharmaceuticals and Eli Lilly and Company) caused an average five-pound weight loss over thirty weeks. Liraglutide (Victoza) showed a slightly higher total weight loss in a fifty-two-week trial. Pramlintide acetate (Symlin) also causes weight loss for many people. However, weight loss is considered a side effect, not an indication for use, in both of these drugs.

FACT

If you or someone you know is at risk for developing type 2 diabetes, getting fit can help cut the risk. The Diabetes Prevention Trial found that minor lifestyle changes, including just thirty minutes of exercise daily, cut the risk of developing type 2 diabetes in high-risk subjects by 58 percent.

People with type 2 diabetes who switch to insulin injections to achieve better control over their blood sugars can also find themselves gaining weight. If you have type 2 and are already overweight or obese, weight gain can increase your insulin resistance, which in turn will increase your insulin dose requirement. It's essential to talk to your doctor about possible adjustments to treatment before you find yourself in a vicious cycle of insulin resistance and weight gain.

If you continue to gain weight or become concerned about the weight you've gained so far, a strategy session with your doctor and dietitian is in order. They may be able to recommend dietary and insulin adjustments that can help bring your unwanted weight gain to a halt. Sometimes a switch to a different insulin type or an insulin pump can help you to get a handle on weight fluctuations.

ALERT

A number of diabetes medications can have initial unpleasant side effects related to weight loss. Metformin is notorious for its gastrointestinal side effects, and Byetta and Amylin often cause nausea. Fortunately, these side effects frequently disappear with time.

Weight Loss and Type 2 Diabetes

The Diabetes Prevention Program (DPP) proved that even modest weight loss can prevent or delay the onset of type 2 diabetes in overweight at-risk adults. But what about people who already have the disease? The news is good for you as well. Weight loss can reduce your need for medication and insulin, improve your cardiovascular health, and, best of all, it will make you feel good about yourself.

FACT

One-year results from the Look AHEAD (Action for Health in Diabetes) study found that type 2 diabetes participants who lost an average of 8.6 percent of their body weight achieved significant cardiovascular and glycemic benefits—including a mean A1C reduction from 7.2 to 6.6.

Weight and Insulin Resistance

Precisely how excess fat promotes insulin resistance isn't yet entirely clear, but it is thought that stored fat releases certain proteins and/or enzymes that act on muscle and liver cells to impair the way that they "read" insulin signals to process glucose. In addition, research has found that the "apple-shaped" body (central abdominal obesity) associated with insulin resistance and type 2 diabetes contains fat with unique properties. Specifically, this type of visceral abdominal fat sheds more free fatty acids, which can elevate triglyceride levels, and is associated with higher insulin levels that promote further fat storage. Paring down abdominal fat will have the double benefit of both increasing insulin sensitivity and decreasing triglyceride levels in people with type 2 diabetes.

Shedding Smart

First, you need a plan that dovetails with your diabetes management program. Book a date with your dietitian so you can strategize on meal plans that promote weight loss. Talk to your doctor before embarking on any new exercise plan so he can assess your heart health and give your workout his official stamp of approval.

If you have diabetic complications or other health issues that affect your mobility, an exercise physiologist and/or physical therapist may be able to get you on track with a low-impact or adaptive exercise program.

Set Realistic Goals

Many people abandon perfectly good weight-loss programs before they even lace up their sneakers. Why? Because Americans live in a world filled with fast food, instant messaging, and five-second glucose meters, anything without a quick payoff goes against the grain of the instant gratification ethic. While it would be nice to "drop inches in days!" as the miracle ads proclaim, the truth is that weight loss is a slow and (hopefully) steady process that takes time and commitment.

Setting realistic weight-loss goals for yourself can be a good motivator. Gradual weight loss is usually the safest method. A diet that cuts your normal calorie consumption (for your weight) by 500 to 1,000 will encourage weight loss. So will burning 500 to 1,000 calories each day with exercise. Your best bet is to strike a balance between the two, and make exercise—be it team sports, cycling, or walking—something you enjoy. Making a long-term healthy lifestyle change is essential to keeping the pounds off once they're gone.

Aim Low

If you wear a misses size 14 and you blow a bundle on a designer size 8 dress as motivation, you'll probably end up feeling guilty, frustrated, and angry if you aren't slinking around in it a month later. You'll do much better setting small, achievable targets for yourself. If you must try the new-clothes strategy, go down a size at a time.

Because weight loss can be a long and bumpy road, you'll find your enthusiasm waning occasionally. Try these strategies to stay inspired and on track:

- **Compete and commiserate.** Set weight-loss goals along with a friend or spouse. A little friendly competition can be just the motivation you need, and you'll also have someone to call and talk you down when that ice cream sundae just won't stop calling your name.
- **Reward yourself.** Find nonedible indulgences to tell yourself "good job!"
- **Scale back.** Don't weigh yourself obsessively. Once a week—at the same time of day—is all you need to monitor your progress.
- **Take baby steps.** Everyone starts somewhere. Even a walk around the block is better than sitting on the couch wishing you had the stamina to go on a bike ride with your kids.

What Doesn't Work

There are also plenty of weight-loss strategies that are guaranteed to backfire:

- **Skipping meals.** Forgoing food completely is hard on your diabetes control, may cause a hypoglycemic episode, and will probably only be effective in making you eat twice as much at the next meal.
- **Skipping meds.** Purposely skipping your shots is dangerous. Insulin omission is not an effective method of weight loss and can trigger life-threatening highs.
- **Dieting without exercise, or vice versa.** Decreasing calories and increasing activity are both required for successful weight loss.

- **Perpetual procrastination.** Waiting for a "better time" to start a weight-loss plan won't make it any easier, and it can quite possibly make the task harder. Stop waiting for tomorrow, and begin today.

Mind over Matter

Losing weight with diabetes means you have two challenges to conquer: learning what and how to eat for optimal blood glucose control, and breaking away from bad overeating habits. Eating emotionally rather than in response to hunger cues is at the root of many weight problems. Examine what your "eating triggers" are. Do you use food as a reward, a comfort, a social tool, or simply a release from boredom?

The first step in breaking these habits is recognizing them, and then coming up with positive substitutions. Make a reward something that feeds your soul rather than your stomach—a few hours with a good book or a weekend getaway with someone special. Try to come up with ways to socialize that aren't focused on food. Meet at a coffeehouse rather than a restaurant, or gather at the park to play football or Frisbee rather than spending another afternoon as armchair quarterbacks. Above all, practice mindful eating. Have meals and snacks away from the television and other distractions that make it too easy to gobble up twice as much as you intended. Enjoy your food, and then move on. Fortunately, good diabetes management encourages mindful eating.

ALERT

Try to rely more on the way you feel than on the tale of the tape. If the scale tells you you're losing weight more slowly than you'd like, but you're feeling energetic and positive about your weight-loss efforts, then you're doing fine. Again, weight loss is not a quick process.

The Low-Carb Conundrum

Low-carb diets are the subject of heated debate in the diabetes community. At first glance, the issue seems cut-and-dried. Carbohydrates cause blood sugar to rise, so wouldn't a low-carb diet automatically be beneficial for someone with diabetes? But low-carb also goes against everything the USDA and nutritionists have been saying for the past several decades—that the vast majority of your calories (45 to 65 percent) should come from carbohydrates.

The Pros and Cons

It's an undisputed fact that dietary carbohydrates increase blood sugar levels. Minimize your carb intake, and you'll minimize increases in blood glucose. So low-carb appears to have a logical, though still disputed, place in diabetes management. But what about low-carb for weight loss? In a nutshell, low-carb proponents blame weight gain on high insulin levels, which can promote fat storage. Since insulin release is triggered by dietary carbohydrates, the reasoning is that too many carbs means too much glucose, which in turn leads to high levels of circulating insulin (hyperinsulinemia), which cause fat storage and weight gain. This hyperinsulinemia can also lead to inflammation in the body that can worsen insulin resistance over time.

QUESTION

I keep seeing "net carbs" on different foods at the grocery store. What does that mean?
"Net carbs" and "effective carbs" are marketing terms coined by food manufacturers. In theory, "net carbs" are those that impact blood sugar. That means that the manufacturer has subtracted carbs from ingredients like sugar alcohols, glycerin, and fiber from the total carbohydrate grams. So proceed with caution, and test your blood sugar before and after eating to see if that "net carb" number really works for you.

The ADA does not endorse the Atkins program and similar low-carb plans for long-term diabetes control, saying that the high-fat and high-protein content in these diets can be dangerous for people with diabetes who are already at risk for coronary artery disease. The other issue with low-carb diets is their high-protein content, which can be tough on the kidneys of people who have advanced kidney disease.

Nonetheless, many people swear by such programs—saying that a low-carb diet has given them their blood sugar control back. Most successful low-carb plans require dieters to pay attention to calories as well as carbs; too much fat can add too many calories to your diet, and without calorie reduction, weight loss simply won't occur. If you do decide to give low-carb dieting a try, discuss it with your doctor first, and then work with your registered dietitian on a customized plan for you.

The Research

In 2003, the *New England Journal of Medicine* published two important controlled clinical trials that put low-carb to the test among people with significant weight and health problems. One study found that obese participants with diabetes who were restricted to 30 grams of carbs daily achieved greater weight loss, maintained better glucose control, and cut triglyceride levels more than their counterparts who were put on a low-fat diet. The second trial had a smaller study population but came to similar conclusions. However, the authors also concluded that the difference in these health benefits between low-fat and low-carb became insignificant after the first six months.

FACT

In 2008, the American Diabetes Association issued its first-ever formal clinical recognition of the potential benefit of low-carb dieting, stating in its nutrition guidelines that low-carb diets "may be effective in the short term" (i.e., up to two years) for weight loss.

Subsequent trials have also revealed weight loss and health benefits to low-carb eating. One of these was the A to Z Weight Loss Study, which put four popular weight-loss diets—Atkins, Ornish, LEARN, and the Zone—in a head-to-head competition. Results published in the *Journal of the American Medical Association* found that twelve months into the study, those study subjects on the low-carb Atkins program had lost the most weight and achieved the biggest health benefits (in terms of improved cholesterol profiles and lower fasting insulin and glucose levels), as compared to those on the higher-carb alternative diets.

However, a meta-analysis of studies of low-carb versus low-fat diets for weight loss published in the *Archives of Internal Medicine* concluded that while low-carb diets were at least as effective as low-fat diets for weight loss, they were associated with unfavorable changes in total and LDL (bad) cholesterol levels. On a more positive note, the study also found that low-carb dieting was associated with favorable changes in triglyceride and HDL (or good) cholesterol levels.

Further long-term, large-scale trials are needed to analyze the risks and potential pluses of low-carb in diabetes treatment. In the meantime, the bottom line is that current research acknowledges the benefits of limiting carbohydrates for weight loss and diabetes control. If you have high LDL or total cholesterol, your doctor should monitor your cholesterol levels carefully if you choose to go on a low-carb diet.

Glycemic Index Diets

The glycemic index (GI), the subject of many bestselling diet books, is another dietary hot potato. The GI focuses on the choice of carbs rather than carb restriction. Low-GI foods raise blood glucose levels at a slow and steady rate, promoting weight loss by discouraging blood sugar spikes and high circulating levels of insulin. The GI has a solid foundation in science and many faithful followers, but using the GI requires some dedicated math skills and an even more dedicated patient.

ALERT

Most fad diets are just that—a fleeting fancy. At best, they drain your wallet and your self-confidence; at their worst, they can be hazardous to your health. Any diet that claims dramatic results in days or a few weeks, or that relies on "testimonials" instead of hard science, is probably destined for failure.

Since glycemic index information isn't something you'll find on the nutrition facts label of packaged foods, there's a lot of homework involved in becoming familiar with what is low, and high, on the scale. Fortunately pocket-sized reference books and smartphone apps make things a bit easier for those that want to give it a try.

Weight-Loss Drugs

When diet and exercise just aren't doing the job for whatever reason, there are other options. The weight-loss medication Xenical (orlistat) shows promise in treating obesity. In clinical trials, Xenical produced a 5 percent or higher weight loss in 72 percent of subjects over a period of six months.

In 2007, the FDA cleared an over-the-counter version of orlistat, called alli, for commercial sale. The drug is the same as the prescription version, but comes in dosages of half the strength (60 mg versus 120 mg) and is accompanied by an online companion behavioral weight-loss program. The ADA recommends that weight-loss medications only be used in patients with a BMI of 27 or higher, and always in conjunction with lifestyle modifications (i.e., diet and exercise).

In June of 2012, the FDA approved Belviq (lorcaserin; from Arena Pharmaceuticals), the first new prescription weight loss drug in over a decade. Belviq works on brain chemistry to increase the feeling of fullness. In trials, Belviq helped patients lose 5 percent or more of their weight when they combined the drug with diet and exercise, and keep that weight off for up to two years. In studies that focused specifically on people with type 2 diabetes, 38 percent of patients taking Belviq achieved similar weight loss percentages and improved blood sugar control.

As this book goes to press, one more new weight loss drug, Qnexa (Vivus), has been endorsed by an FDA advisory panel and awaits final FDA approval. Qnexa is a combination of the appetite-suppressant phentermine and the anti-seizure drug topiramate. The FDA is expected to decide on Qnexa by the end of 2012.

Side Effects

Both Xenical and alli can cause considerably unpleasant gastrointestinal side effects, including cramping, diarrhea, gas, and leakage of oily stools. Eating foods with high fat content will worsen these side effects.

For people with diabetes, the most common side effects from taking Belviq are low blood sugar (hypoglycemia), headache, back pain, cough, and fatigue. Because Belviq increases serotonin levels, people who take drugs that increase serotonin levels or activate serotonin receptors, such as drugs to treat depression and migraine, should be cautious when taking Belviq. Belviq may also cause problems with attention or memory.

Gastric Surgery

Finally, for severely obese people with type 2 diabetes who have been unable to lose weight using traditional means, gastric-bypass or reduction surgery, also called bariatric surgery, may be an option. Only patients with a BMI greater or equal to 35 are typically considered for bariatric surgery.

A number of different types of bariatric surgery are available, including adjustable gastric banding, vertical-banded gastroplasty, Roux-en-Y gastric bypass, and biliopancreatic diversion (with or without a duodenal switch). The first two of these are restrictive surgeries, and work by closing off the majority of the stomach to the digestive process, leaving only a small section to digest food. The latter two are bypass (or malabsorptive) operations, which reroute the digestive flow past part or all of the small intestine to minimize the amount of calories that can be absorbed.

Laparoscopic adjustable banding (also called lap banding) is the most common type of bariatric surgical procedure. As with traditional adjustable gastric banding, a portion of the stomach is banded off with a device that can be inflated or deflated to change the size of the stomach pouch as required. However, lap banding uses a minimally invasive laparoscopic procedure that involves small incisions and the use of surgical cameras to position the band. This technique minimizes both recovery time and the risk of complications (as compared to traditional bariatric surgery).

ALERT

While laparoscopic banding surgery carries fewer surgical risks and a shorter recovery time than other gastric surgeries, it isn't an option for everyone. If you are severely obese, have significant heart or lung problems, or have had previous stomach surgery, you may require traditional surgery versus laparoscopic.

Bariatric surgery carries the same risks of infection and hemorrhage as any major surgery, plus a high rate of related complications; up to 20 percent of people who have bariatric surgery have to undergo follow-up operations to fix abdominal hernias or other problems. Gallstones are also a risk because of the rapid weight loss that occurs following the operation. And because some types of surgery bypass the small intestine, where a great deal of nutrient absorption takes place, approximately 30 percent of patients end up with deficiencies of certain vitamins and minerals (a condition that can usually be corrected with supplementation).

Recent research shows that certain bariatric surgeries improve blood sugar control independently of the weight loss they facilitate. In other words, blood sugar improvements occur postsurgery, before significant weight loss has occurred. While scientists are still researching the mechanisms behind this, they believe it is related to the changes in levels of gut hormones that gastric bypass and banding triggers.

Keeping It Off

Weight maintenance can be a lifelong challenge. Sometimes you can't control the situations that put the pounds back on. Illness or injury can hamper your exercise efforts or required drug therapy may promote weight gain. When health conditions cause weight gain, sometimes the only thing you can do is wait it out and get back on your program when things resolve.

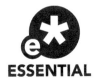

ESSENTIAL

Keep a diary of your weight-loss progress. It can help you become familiar with the things that trigger weight gain and slip-ups for you, and make you much less likely to fall prey to them the next time around.

You can avoid slipping back into old habits like emotional eating, exercise avoidance, or plain old procrastination. In fact, having diabetes may make it easier for you to stay on track, because you have to pay attention to your body by default. And when you do stumble, remember that it isn't the end of the world. You're simply learning another lesson about yourself and your health that will benefit your emotional management of diabetes in the long run.

CHAPTER 11

In Case of Emergency

One minute you're fine; the next you are dizzy, shaky, and disoriented. Blood sugar highs and lows—the literal peaks and valleys of diabetes—are perhaps the scariest part of the disease. While everyone living with diabetes strives for blood sugar balance, occasional hyperglycemia (blood sugar highs) and hypoglycemia (blood sugar lows) are virtually unavoidable. Preparation, prevention, and patience are the keys to getting through these episodes and staying in control of your diabetes.

Hypoglycemic Episodes

Hypoglycemia, also known as an insulin reaction, a blood sugar low, or a hypo, can hit hard and fast, leaving you shaky, confused, and scared. While many people with type 2 diabetes do not experience lows, if you take insulin or certain classes of type 2 diabetes medications (i.e., sulfonylureas, meglitinides) you are at risk and should learn how to treat them.

Everyone has differing levels of sensitivity to blood sugar drops. One person may start to feel "funny" at 70 mg/dl (3.9 mmol/l), while another can drop considerably lower before sensing that something is wrong. Some people can also experience a condition known as hypoglycemic unawareness, a condition in which the body no longer reacts to low blood glucose levels with the usual symptoms. Your doctor will help you establish what reading is too low for you. Low episodes in patients taking insulin or one of the diabetes medications described above are typically caused by one of three things:

1. Too much insulin or diabetes medication (sulfonylureas or meglitinides)
2. Too little food
3. Exercise without enough carbohydrates

When it comes to dealing effectively with hypoglycemia, you need to be prepared, practice prevention, and exercise patience. Carry a fast-acting sugar or carb at all times; test often and treat at the first sign of a low; and don't panic. If you overreact and, say, drink two liters of soda, you can easily end up on a roller coaster of highs and lows. Read on for the most effective way to treat a low quickly without causing blood sugar rebounds.

Signs and Symptoms

Blood sugar lows are dangerous because the brain needs glucose to function properly. A severe, untreated low can cause a loss of consciousness. Other symptoms of hypoglycemia include the following:

- Shakiness (trembling hands, etc.)
- Dizziness or lightheadedness
- Headache

- Hunger
- Heart palpitations
- Sudden sweating
- Clammy or pale skin
- Irritability or unexplained mood swings
- Confusion or disorientation

Treating a Hypo

Once your blood glucose meter has confirmed a low, take action immediately. The rule of thumb for treating a low blood sugar is to take 15 grams of a fast-acting carb, wait fifteen minutes, and test again. Good, quick carb options include glucose tablets, a half glass of orange juice, or glucose gel. If you're looking for a more tasty option for treatment, you can try tubes of decorative cake frosting or sugary chewable candy like Sweet Tarts, Spree, Smarties, and Life Savers, which are also effective and portable choices (candies used to treat hypos should be chewed and not sucked). Check the labels for carb amounts so you aren't over- or under-treating your lows.

If your levels are still too low after testing the second time, have another 15 grams of carbs, wait fifteen minutes, and test again. Anytime you don't have your glucose monitor with you to check your blood but feel the symptoms of a hypo, trust your instincts and assume your glucose levels are low.

FACT

Fat can delay the absorption of sugar, so if you're treating a low, doughnuts, chocolate bars, and ice cream aren't the best choices. While these foods will do in a pinch, they will take longer to bring glucose back up. Instead, keep a roll of glucose tablets or a tube of glucose gel in your purse, car, and desk, and you'll always be prepared.

It is possible to lose consciousness and have a seizure when blood glucose levels drop extremely low. For this reason, it's always a good idea to have someone nearby and accessible (e.g., spouse, friend, coworker, or teacher) who knows exactly what to do in case of a hypoglycemic episode.

If you are still conscious, a companion can assist you in taking a fast-acting carb by mouth. This should not be attempted if you are unconscious because of the risk of choking. If you lose consciousness, an injection of the hormone glucagon should be administered; if glucagon is not available, someone should call 911 immediately.

How Glucagon Works

Glucagon stimulates the liver to convert stored glycogen back into glucose. A glucagon kit contains a syringe and a vial of powdered glucagon. The fluid in the prefilled syringe is mixed with the powder immediately before use, drawn into the syringe, and then injected like insulin into a large muscle, such as the thigh or buttock.

Glucagon is available by prescription only. Your doctor or CDE (certified diabetes educator) can give you a quick lesson on how and when to use it. Glucagon may not work as effectively to treat a low that was caused by drinking alcohol. It will also not work if an insufficient amount of glycogen is available in the liver (such as in cases of malnutrition). Glucagon can cause nausea and possible vomiting, so you should let whomever you instruct in its use know that they should place you on your side if you are given glucagon and are still unconscious.

ESSENTIAL

Always store the instructions for your glucagon injection with the syringe. Even with the best preparation, people can forget what they're supposed to be doing in an emotionally charged situation. Make sure you periodically check the expiration date on your glucagon kit, so it is always ready—just in case.

Night Hypos

Even the very idea of having a low in the middle of the night is frightening. Will you wake up? Will your partner wake up? If your blood sugar levels are below 100 mg/dl at bedtime, you are more likely to experience a low during the night. Fortunately, with a little planning and treatment adjustments, the problem is usually remedied relatively easily.

Nighttime lows are most common in people taking insulin. Typically, a person pumps out less glucose between midnight and 3 A.M. because the body is at rest and simply doesn't need it. If your insulin peaks during the time when glucose production is unusually low, a hypo could result. Exercise could be the culprit of a hypo if you work out intensely in the evening. Try to work out earlier in the day, or talk to your doctor about adjusting your insulin dose before working out to accommodate the natural drop in blood sugar that exercise produces.

A bedtime snack can often ward off middle-of-the-night drops in some people. The snack should contain protein, which will lengthen the release of the carbohydrate. If you are on insulin and nighttime lows persist despite treatment adjustments, an insulin pump (which can be programmed to avoid highs and lows even while you sleep) or changes in your insulin therapy may be options.

If you're experiencing night lows, and have not yet found a treatment approach that works well for you, it's a good idea to set your alarm to wake you up for a test several times during the night. Make sure you have glucose tablets or another quick carb on your nightstand just in case you need it. Track the testing info and review it with your doctor to try to find a pattern to your lows.

Sometimes lows that occur while you sleep cause morning fasting blood sugar levels (before breakfast) to be elevated. This phenomenon, known as the Somogyi effect or rebound, happens when the body starts producing glucagon and epinephrine in response to a low. These hormones signal the liver to convert glycogen to glucose, and the result is high blood sugars upon waking. If your blood glucose is elevated at your first morning test, there's a possibility it's due to an undetected nighttime low. However, it may also be a result of the dawn phenomenon, which is a morning high caused by the natural release of blood glucose in the early-morning hours.

Hypoglycemic Unawareness

Sometimes, people who have had diabetes for many years develop hypoglycemic unawareness—blood glucose lows that they don't know about because they don't show any symptoms. This may be caused in part by damage to the sympathetic nervous system (called autonomic neuropathy), in which the typical involuntary reactions to low blood sugars—such as sweating and flushing—don't occur. For some people with this condition, a loss of consciousness is their first and only sign that their blood glucose has dipped dangerously low.

QUESTION

Are there any devices that can wake me up from a low at night?
Today's continuous blood glucose monitoring systems have alarms that can be set to go off if your blood sugar drops too low or climbs too high. There are also several devices on the market, which are worn like a wristwatch, that sound an alarm when they detect perspiration or a drop in skin temperature—two signs of a hypo.

If you experience lows frequently, you're more likely to develop hypoglycemic unawareness. This can be an unintended side effect of a regimen of intensive blood glucose control. These patients are three times more likely to experience hypoglycemic unawareness than those on a nonintensive treatment program. And if you have a hypo, your risk of having yet another low is higher for up to two days following the episode. If you're trying to keep your blood sugars in tight control, you have a fine line to walk, and you might sometimes end up in a vicious cycle of low after low. Eventually, hypoglycemic unawareness may result. This is another reason that frequent testing of your blood sugar levels is so important.

If you develop hypoglycemic unawareness while on an intensive control program, your doctor will probably recommend increasing your target blood glucose levels slightly to avoid dangerous lows. Some clinical studies have shown that, in some patients, loosening control to allow blood glucose levels to run slightly high for two to three weeks can restore hypoglycemia awareness.

If you have hypoglycemic unawareness, blood glucose awareness training may also be an option for you. Frequent monitoring, increased awareness of hypo triggers, and recognition of some of the subtler signs of a low are the focus of this type of training. If you experience blood glucose readings of 50 mg/dl or less without any signs of hypoglycemia, let your doctor know immediately. It is probably a sign of hypoglycemic unawareness, and some adjustments to treatment may be in order.

Several studies have found that moderate intake of caffeine may be useful in heightening sensitivity to symptoms of blood glucose lows in those patients with hypoglycemic unawareness. Be sure to check with your doctor before increasing your caffeine intake, as too much caffeine can have negative consequences, particularly if you have high blood pressure.

High Blood Sugar Emergencies

On the other end of the blood sugar spectrum is hyperglycemia, or blood sugar highs. The occasional high blood sugar won't hurt you, and is in fact fairly hard to avoid. But if those elevated blood sugar levels are allowed to continue and aren't managed properly, they will damage your body and put you at risk for a long list of diabetic complications.

It's also very important for you to become familiar with the signs and symptoms of a high blood sugar emergency. If you become ill or injured, the stress on your body can raise your blood sugar levels to dangerous levels. This can result in one of two life-threatening conditions—hyperosmolar hyperglycemia syndrome or diabetic ketoacidosis.

Hyperosmolar Hyperglycemia Syndrome

Extremely high blood sugar levels can lead to hyperosmolar hyperglycemia syndrome (also called hyperglycemic hyperosmolar nonketotic coma or syndrome or HHNS). This condition is most common in older adults with type 2 who are also experiencing other health issues, such as illness or injury, that drive up their blood sugar levels.

Sometimes, people who develop HHNS are on drugs that raise their blood glucose levels, or become dehydrated due to diuretic medications or illness. HHNS also commonly occurs in elderly patients with previously undiagnosed diabetes. Having impaired kidney function may increase your risk of developing HHNS. HHNS can occur at blood glucose levels about

600 mg/dl (33.3 mmol/l). At diagnosis, plasma glucose levels are usually much higher in diabetic ketoacidosis, or DKA (near 1000 mg/dl, or 55.5 mmol/l).

In HHNS, hyperglycemia occurs without ketosis (the formation of ketone bodies that happens in DKA, described later in this chapter). Extreme dehydration causes a dangerous drop in blood pressure and has the potential to cause cardiovascular collapse. There is a high mortality rate associated with HHNS.

HHNS may take days or weeks to build up to a crisis point. If you are ill and your glucose levels are persistently above 240 mg/dl, even if you test negative for ketones, you should still call your doctor for further advice. If you exhibit any of the signs of HHNS along with elevated blood sugar levels, call your doctor immediately or go to the nearest emergency care facility.

Possible symptoms of HHNS include:

- Frequent urination
- Excessive thirst
- Nausea and vomiting
- High fever
- Weight loss
- Dehydration
- Weakness, especially on one side of the body
- Seizures
- Hallucinations
- Confusion, unconsciousness, or coma

To treat a person with HHNS, saline is administered intravenously to restore fluid balance to the bloodstream. Electrolytes may also be given. Insulin therapy may or may not be needed. Finding out the root cause or event that triggered the HHNS is key to preventing its recurrence.

Diabetic Ketoacidosis (DKA)

Diabetic ketoacidosis (DKA) can develop when glucose levels climb to 250 mg/dl (13.9 mmol/l) or higher and ketones are present in the blood or urine. As opposed to HHNS, which can have a slow and subtle onset, DKA escalates quickly. While DKA is more common in type 1 diabetes patients, it can also occur in people with type 2. DKA happens when, in the absence of sufficient insulin (which enables the body to use glucose for energy), the body starts to break down fat for energy. Fat metabolism causes ketone bodies to form, which throws off the acid balance in the bloodstream. Meanwhile, the liver continues to pump out more and more glucose, and so blood glucose climbs higher and higher. The result is ketoacidosis.

When the body is under a severe degree of stress, hyperglycemia and DKA may occur. Infection, injury, surgical procedures, and even a simple cold or flu are all known offenders in causing blood glucose to rise. Sometimes people skip their insulin or medication because they are ill, which then boosts blood glucose even higher. Dehydration caused by vomiting and diarrhea can also worsen blood glucose levels.

ALERT

Never skip a dose of medication just because you are ill. Illness usually causes blood sugars to climb, and skipping your meds can make the problem worse. In many cases, you may require more insulin when you are ill. Talk to your doctor about a "sick-day plan" for your medications and/or insulin dose.

Often, the symptoms of DKA are initially ignored because many closely resemble the flu or a viral infection. Because the flu itself causes blood sugars to rise and can trigger DKA complicates matters further. This is why frequent testing and staying on your treatment schedule is so important when you are ill. Symptoms of DKA include the following:

- Fruity smell on the breath (from acetone)
- Nausea
- Vomiting
- Fatigue
- Muscle aches and stiffness
- Abdominal pain
- Extreme thirst and frequent urination
- Rapid breathing or difficulty breathing
- Mental confusion
- Unconsciousness or, in extreme cases, coma

A rare but potentially fatal complication of DKA is cerebral edema (swelling of the brain). Signs of cerebral edema include severe headache, irritability, drowsiness, and confusion.

Diabetic ketoacidosis should always be treated by a health care professional. Treatment consists of lowering blood glucose levels with insulin and restoring fluid and electrolyte balance with oral fluids or intravenous saline. In some cases, potassium or other electrolytes may also be administered intravenously. If the underlying cause of DKA is illness or infection, then that illness should be treated appropriately to prevent a recurrence of DKA.

When to Test for Ketones

If your blood glucose levels are over 240 mg/dl (13.3 mmol/l), then you should test for ketones. Ketone testing is particularly important when you are ill. Home urine tests, which consist of reagent strips that can be dipped in a urine sample and checked against a diagnostic color chart, are easy to perform and are an excellent tool for avoiding DKA. There are also combination blood glucose and ketone meters available in the United States that are useful for home testing. Ask your health care provider if home ketone monitoring is appropriate for you.

FACT

Many over-the-counter and prescription medications can raise blood glucose levels, including steroids, atypical antipsychotics, and glucocorticoids. Drugs that induce dehydration can also cause dangerous hyperglycemic episodes. Before taking any new medications, talk to your doctor about potential side effects.

High-Risk Situations

Several situations can cause blood glucose levels to nose-dive or skyrocket. Being prepared for them, when and if they occur, is the best way to avoid the possible highs and lows.

Sick Days

Being ill is a big risk factor for high blood glucose levels. If your doctor hasn't discussed it with you already, you should ask him about a sick-day plan. A sick-day plan is simply a course of action to take if you develop the flu or another mild illness. Here are some typical guidelines to follow when you are sick:

- **Keep eating and drinking.** Have plenty of nonperishable food and drinks on hand that are easy on the tummy, including sugar-free Jell-O, broth soups, saltine crackers, low-sugar fruit juice, and sugar-free pudding. Drink plenty of water and fluids to avoid dehydration.
- **Stock up the medicine cabinet.** In addition to your glucose meter, you should always have ketone-testing supplies on hand, and basics like a thermometer and medications to treat diarrhea and vomiting. Talk to your doctor about recommendations for the latter.
- **Stay in touch.** Discuss guidelines with your doctor about when you should call him (e.g., if your blood glucose reaches a certain landmark, or if you can't keep food down, or if you exhibit specific symptoms). When in doubt, always pick up the phone.
- **Test often.** Stating the obvious—you'll need to test frequently so that you are aware of dangerous highs early.
- **Don't skip your meds.** Keep taking both insulin and oral medications. If they do not bring down your blood sugar adequately, call your doctor to discuss increasing the dose.

Drinking Alcohol

When you drink alcohol, your liver shuts down its regular glycogen storage and glucose production operation, opting instead to concentrate on clearing the alcohol from your body. The result can be hypoglycemia, which can occur either while you're drinking or hours afterward, while your liver continues to clear alcohol from the bloodstream. For this reason, you should always eat when you drink, and be on the lookout for symptoms of a low.

Be sure to assess any mixed drinks for "hidden" calories and sugar from fruit juices or mixes (and work them into your overall meal plan). A snack before bed is also important if you've indulged to ward off overnight lows. And when you've been drinking, it's always a good idea to set your alarm to awaken you for a middle-of- the-night blood test for the same reason.

If you choose to drink alcohol, it is absolutely essential that you have a non-drinking friend with you who knows how to recognize the symptoms of hypoglycemia and how to treat them appropriately. Because alcohol can so easily impair judgment, this friend should be someone you can trust not to drink.

Even if you choose to abstain or have only one drink, but attend a function where the alcohol is flowing freely, it's important to have a designated nondrinking buddy who knows what to look out for. Some of the symptoms of a low—confusion, mood swings, and incoherence—can easily be mistaken for intoxication by others (especially if they've had a few themselves) and not treated appropriately.

Medications

Certain medications can cause highs or lows. Whenever you get a new prescription, ask your doctor about its potential to affect your blood glucose levels and what adjustments you can make to your treatment to avoid a blood sugar emergency. And for the same reason, never take supplements or herbal remedies without consulting your doctor first.

Make sure you are never caught without your diabetes medication. Always get your insulin and oral drug prescriptions filled well before you run out. If you ever find yourself in the position of not being able to afford your medication, call your doctor and explain your circumstances. In many cases, she may be able to offer you drug samples to get you through a particularly difficult time. She may also be able to prescribe a less expensive generic or alternative drug.

ESSENTIAL

Several patient assistance programs are available through major pharmaceutical manufacturers that offer drugs to those who need them at a reduced rate or free of charge.

Buddy System

Embarrassed, ashamed, self-conscious, guilty, alone—do any of these describe the way you're feeling about having diabetes? First, realize that you aren't to blame for having this disease. These feelings are a natural part of coming to terms with your diagnosis. It may take some time to overcome them completely, but in the meantime, you need to get past them enough to let the people around you know you need their help.

As of the writing of this book, there were nearly 26 million people living with diabetes in the United States. That makes the odds pretty darn good that at least a few of your coworkers, neighbors, friends, and family have already been touched by the disease. With that in mind, they may already know a lot about diabetes; then again, they may be sorely in need of some accurate and current diabetes education. Either way, you only have to share the basics of handling an emergency.

First, have a "buddy" (or two or three) at each place you frequent regularly, such as work, the gym or playing field, class, church, and so on. Let your buddies know (and give them access to) where you keep your basic supplies (i.e., meter, fast-acting glucose, and glucagon kit), and provide them with instructions on administering glucagon. Most of the glucagon kits on the market include illustrated instructions that will make it easier for your buddy to give you an injection.

ALERT

When educating friends, family, and coworkers about potential emergency situations, make sure they understand the difference between insulin and glucagon. Because both medications are injected, they may easily be confused, a situation that could have life-threatening consequences if you were to lose consciousness and be treated with the wrong drug.

These basic guidelines can give them direction for assisting you. Customize them to your own particular blood sugar highs and lows:

• If I look ill or am acting strange, ask me if I'm okay and suggest that I check my blood sugars.

- If I test low (less than 70 mg/dl or as indicated by a low alarm on my meter) and am still conscious, help me to eat or drink some glucose tablets, juice, or other fast-acting sugars.
- If I test extremely high (over 240 mg/dl or as indicated by a high alarm on my meter), and I lose consciousness or am incoherent, call 911 immediately.
- If I test low and lose consciousness, do not try to feed me. Call 911 immediately and administer a glucagon injection.
- If I haven't tested or you don't know what my blood sugar levels are and I lose consciousness, never try to feed me or give me insulin. Instead, call 911 immediately.

Medical Identification

Even if you've got a buddy with you at all times, it's important that you always carry medical identification in case you need to be treated by medical personnel. Wearing some visible form of ID at all times is the best way to ensure that you will get proper treatment should a blood sugar emergency cause you to lose consciousness among strangers.

It may be tempting to take off your ID at the gym or before a run. Don't. During (and following) exercise is a high-risk time for hypoglycemia. The same goes for social events and parties with alcohol. Living with diabetes means that blood sugar lows and highs can strike any time. Don't be caught unprepared.

The Options

When you're shopping for a medical ID, keep these elements in mind:

- It must be noticeable—this is the most important criterion for a good ID.
- It must be comfortable—otherwise you won't wear it.
- It should be durable enough to stand up to sun, surf, and whatever other elements you may encounter.
- It should be comprehensive—make sure it lists all pertinent medical information.
- It should be stylish. Make sure you like it, or, again, you won't wear it.

Your ID should indicate that you have diabetes. If you take insulin, it should say that as well, along with any drug allergies you may have. Your tag will let paramedics and other health care providers know that they should test your blood glucose before treating you.

What Works and What Doesn't

Some people don't like to shout out "I have diabetes!" and so they opt for less intrusive means of identification, like a key chain or a wallet card. Unfortunately, being subtle doesn't do you a whole lot of good in an emergency situation. If you lose consciousness, the only person who may go immediately for your wallet or your car keys would be a mugger or carjacker. A medical alert bracelet, pendant, or watchband is much more likely to be noticed for the right reason.

ESSENTIAL

Always test your blood glucose before you drive—make it a habit. If it's too low, treat it and wait for the subsequent rise before turning on the ignition. Even the slightest lapse in concentration can have serious repercussions behind the wheel of a car. Driving with a blood glucose low can be just as dangerous as drinking and driving.

Most medical IDs are marked with a caduceus, a winged staff entwined with snakes, which is the Greek symbol for medicine. Today's medical ID products are available in a wide variety of configurations, including watch tags, bracelets, pendants, sports bands, shoelace tags, clip-on ID cards, custom-made gemstone jewelry, and even temporary tattoos. Products like shoelace tags (which are worn securely at the toe end of the laces) are good choices for young children who may not like to wear bracelets or pendants.

Emergency Response Services

If you have a complicated medical history, or simply want to have more peace of mind regarding treatment of your diabetes in an emergency, you can invest in a subscription to an emergency response service like Medic-Alert. These companies store your detailed medical information in a database, then issue you a medical identification engraved with both your medical condition and their toll-free number. When hospital or emergency personnel call the number, your information can be relayed to them.

QUESTION

I am considering getting a tattoo that says I have diabetes to keep myself safe. Are there any risks?
The main risks are infection and slow healing. Ask your doctor what she thinks. If your diabetes is in good control and you have no other complicating skin or nerve conditions, she may give you the green light. Just remember that if you're using the tattoo as a medical identifier, place it somewhere where it will be seen by anyone giving you medical aid, like your wrist.

If you aren't willing or able to make an investment in a service like MedicAlert, some standard ID products feature compartments for storing more extensive written medical information. Just remember that in a crisis situation, time is of the essence. Emergency medical personnel will see a standard ID first when they check your pulse, so your best bet is to wear a medical ID bracelet or necklace that clearly states that you have diabetes.

CHAPTER 12

Diabetes and Your Body

Your body is equipped with 60,000 miles of blood vessels and wired with a whopping 100,000 miles of nerve fibers. A clog here, some corrosion there, and all this hardware suffers from the strain. Diabetes is like a bad tenant who backs up pipes and short-circuits wiring. You may not be able to evict this tenant, but with proper maintenance you can do your part to prevent long-term systemic complications.

Heart Health

According to the U.S. Centers for Disease Control (CDC), a staggering 68 percent of people with diabetes over age sixty-five die from heart disease. Yet few people with diabetes are aware of their increased cardiovascular risks.

Bringing blood sugar, blood pressure, and LDL cholesterol levels down is the best way to combat diabetes-related cardiovascular complications. The National Diabetes Education Program (NDEP) and the Department of Health and Human Services (HHS) recommend following the "ABCs" of diabetes treatment to maintain optimal heart health.

▼ ABCs OF DIABETES TREATMENT

A	A1C	<7 percent
B	Blood pressure	<130/80 mmHg
C	Cholesterol	LDL <100 mg/dl

For patients with a poor cholesterol profile, dietary adjustments (i.e., lowering intake of saturated fat) and increased exercise are recommended. If these adjustments don't provide sufficient improvement, or if LDL and/or triglyceride levels are significantly elevated to begin with, these patients may be prescribed drugs called statins—such as Crestor (rosuvastatin), Lipitor (atorvastatin), Pravachol (pravastatin), or Zocor (simvastatin). In some cases, your physician may recommend a statin drug as a preventive measure, even if your lipid profiles are normal.

FACT

A study published in 2012 found that deaths attributable to heart disease and stroke dropped 40 percent among people with diabetes from 1997–2006. CDC researchers attribute the decline to improvements in cardiovascular treatment, better diabetes management, more physical activity, and a drop in the number of smokers in this population.

Atherosclerosis and CAD

Atherosclerosis, more commonly known as hardening or clogging of the arteries, is caused by a buildup of fatty material (also called plaque or cholesterol), which restricts blood flow. If arteries become completely blocked, tissue death can occur. For patients with arterial obstructions, medications such as nitroglycerin, beta-blockers, and angiotensin-converting enzyme (ACE) inhibitors may be prescribed.

Blockage to the arteries that feed the heart is called coronary artery disease (CAD). What makes CAD particularly dangerous is that symptoms don't typically appear until vessels are significantly blocked. Symptoms of CAD include the following:

- Chest pain (angina)
- Pain in the left arm or shoulder (referred pain)
- Neck or jaw pain
- Chest tightness or pressure
- Shortness of breath
- Nausea
- Perspiration
- Irregular heartbeat (arrhythmia)

ESSENTIAL

In those at risk, an aspirin a day may keep heart disease away. The ADA recommends that adult men and women with a history of or risk factors for CAD, peripheral vascular disease (PVD), stroke, or heart attack take a daily dose of 75 to 162 milligrams of coated aspirin. Aspirin therapy is not recommended for those who have aspirin allergy, some liver problems, or bleeding disorders.

An electrocardiogram (ECG), echocardiogram, and/or stress test may be helpful in diagnosing blocked arteries. If CAD is left untreated or if treatment is ineffective, arteries to the heart may become completely blocked. When blood flow is restricted to the heart, a myocardial infarction (heart attack) may occur. Without oxygen from the blood, the affected area of heart muscle dies.

Symptoms of a heart attack are the same as those described previously for CAD, except the pain is considerably more intense. However, in people with diabetes who suffer from autonomic neuropathy (described later in this chapter), pain symptoms may not be felt at all, resulting in a "silent heart attack."

In cases of stroke or heart attack, where restoring blood flow quickly is critical to prevent tissue death and damage, clot-dissolving or "clot-busting" (fibrinolytic or thrombolytic) drugs may be administered, such as Activase (alteplase) or Retavase (reteplase). These drugs should be given within three hours of the start of stroke symptoms in order to be most effective.

If clot-busting drugs aren't effective, or if too much time has passed, blood clots may be removed by surgical means. Several minimally invasive options are now available that can be used up to eight hours after stroke symptoms occur. One device, the Merci Retriever, consists of a very fine catheter with a corkscrew-shaped device at the end. The catheter is threaded through the large blood vessels of the brain, where the corkscrew wraps itself around the clot. The catheter and the clot are then removed and blood flow is restored. A second catheter system, called the Penumbra, uses suction to remove a clot.

To prevent a recurrence, you may also require an angioplasty, a procedure in which a catheter is inserted into the artery and an attached balloon is expanded to clear the blockage. Often, a device called a stent, which is expanded inside the artery to hold the vessel open, is used. Atherectomy, a procedure that strips fatty blockages out of the artery, may also be performed. Studies have indicated that coronary bypass surgery may have better long-term outcomes than angioplasty for people with diabetes. Bypass involves rerouting the circulation by grafting a healthy piece of artery onto the obstructed blood vessel and around the blockage.

ALERT

Congestive heart failure (CHF) is yet another cardiovascular condition for which people with diabetes are at a higher risk. Symptoms include fluid retention (edema), shortness of breath, heart palpitations, and fatigue. CHF is usually treated with ACE inhibitors, beta-blockers, digoxin, and diuretics.

Peripheral Vascular Disease (PVD)

Like CAD, peripheral vascular disease (also called peripheral arterial disease, or PAD) involves atherosclerosis. Unlike CAD, PVD affects the extremities—most commonly the legs. Signs of PVD include the following:

- Calf and leg cramps or aching, usually when walking, that goes away with rest (intermittent claudication)
- Smooth, shiny, hairless skin on the shins
- Chronically cold feet and legs
- Numb legs or feet
- A bluish or reddish cast to the skin of the feet and/or legs
- Sores or ulcers on the legs that won't heal

The treatment of PVD is similar to that of CAD. Weight loss, cholesterol improvement through diet or drug therapy, appropriate exercise, smoking cessation and medication may all be recommended. Good foot care, important for everyone with diabetes, is especially essential to those people who develop PVD.

Hypertension

Another leading complication of diabetes is hypertension, or high blood pressure. This complication occurs in 67 percent of people with diabetes, and it is also closely linked with both diabetic kidney disease and CAD, which makes it a complex yet critical-to-manage condition.

The ADA recommends that nonpregnant adults with diabetes age eighteen years and older aim for a blood pressure goal of less than 130 mmHg systolic and less than 80 mmHg diastolic (commonly expressed as 130/80 or "130 over 80"). A patient is considered hypertensive if she has a blood pressure reading greater than or equal to 140/90 mmHg.

Weight loss, smoking cessation, exercise, stress management, and dietary adjustments such as lowering sodium and cholesterol intake may all be part of your recommended treatment program if your blood pressure is elevated. All of these treatment goals may be easier to accomplish because they largely align with your diabetes management program goals.

If lifestyle modifications don't bring down your blood pressure, medications such as angiotensin-converting enzyme (ACE) inhibitors, diuretics, and angiotensin receptor blockers (ARBs) are effective options for some people. ACE inhibitors have also been shown to have the added benefit of delaying the progression of kidney disease, and may be a preferred therapy in patients who also have renal impairment. Your doctor can tell you more about these drugs, and if they may be right for you.

Stroke

Another potential cardiovascular complication of diabetes is ischemic stroke. Ischemic stroke occurs when an artery leading to the brain becomes blocked and blood flow is cut off. Symptoms of stroke hit suddenly and include the following:

- Weakness or numbness of the arm, face, or leg (typically one-sided)
- Mental confusion
- Difficulty speaking
- Dizziness and/or problems with balance
- Visual problems
- Severe headache

Because of the complex relationships between diabetes and all the systems of the body, many diabetic complications are interrelated. For example, University of Wisconsin research (the Atherosclerosis Risk in Communities Study) found that middle-aged people who had never experienced a stroke but suffered from retinopathy displayed poorer cognitive function that those who didn't have retinopathy. The finding suggests that cerebral microvascular disease (which is at the root of diabetic retinopathy) may contribute to the development of cognitive impairment, even when stroke doesn't occur.

Neurological Complications

Diabetes is a risk factor for stroke, nerve damage, and cognitive impairment. Stroke is technically a cardiovascular complication caused by a blockage of blood to or a hemorrhage in the brain, but it can cause impairment to memory, vision, speech, movement, and other brain functions in varying degrees of severity.

The most common neurological complications of diabetes are caused by neuropathy, or nerve damage. The exact way that diabetes causes nerve damage is not completely understood yet, but research indicates that over time high levels of blood glucose damage the nerve cells, which unlike other cells don't require an insulin "key" to allow glucose inside them. Researchers have also hypothesized that too much glucose causes depletion of nitric acid, which in turn cuts off blood supply to the nerves.

Peripheral Neuropathy (PN)

Peripheral neuropathy is often called stocking-glove syndrome because it most commonly affects the feet and hands. This condition can be particularly troublesome in the feet because you may develop an injury that you don't notice, and then compound the problem through the simple act of walking. Symptoms of peripheral neuropathy include the following:

- A feeling of "pins and needles"
- Tingling and/or burning sensations
- In some people, pain
- Numbness
- Balance problems (if PN is present in the feet)
- Reflex problems and muscle weakness

FACT

Neuropathies are either diffuse (affecting a wide area or several areas of the body) or focal (affecting a specific place on the body). Most neuropathic conditions related to diabetes are diffuse, including both peripheral and autonomic neuropathy.

The antidepressant medications duloxetine (Cymbalta), amitriptyline, and desipramine may be useful in blocking pain signals, although side effects may be an issue for some patients. Gabapentin (Neurontin) and pregabalin (Lyrica), both anticonvulsant drugs, are also effective treatments for many people with PN and have the additional advantage of having few side effects. A number of studies have also shown promising treatment results with alpha lipoic acid (ALA) treatment, although ALA is not FDA-approved for this particular use at this point in time.

Your doctor may also recommend topical (on the skin) treatment with lidocaine, evening primrose oil, or capsaicin cream (which contains a substance derived from hot peppers that helps to block pain signals). Some anecdotal success has been reported in treating PN with acupuncture and with transcutaneous electronic nerve stimulations (TENS), a procedure that uses electrical waves to block pain signals.

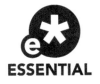

ESSENTIAL

If you have painful peripheral neuropathy and have difficulty sleeping because of it, you may want to invest in a bed cradle. A bed cradle is a device that elevates sheets, blankets, and other bedding above the sensitive spots on feet and legs so you can sleep in comfort but still stay warm.

Anodyne therapy is another PN therapy. It uses flexible pads that contain a series of light-emitting diodes (LEDs) that emit infrared light and energy to penetrate the skin. The light energy and heat is purported to improve circulation and reduce pain. Pads can be placed on the feet, hands, or elsewhere. Published research is conflicted on whether or not anodyne therapy has any lasting therapeutic value in the treatment of PN, and further studies are needed to make this determination.

Autonomic Neuropathy

While many people with diabetes are aware of the signs and symptoms of PN, significantly fewer are educated about, or tested for, autonomic neuropathy. A stealth disorder, autonomic neuropathy short-circuits the nerves that control the sympathetic (autonomic or involuntary) nervous system. Blood pressure, heart rate, perspiration, salivation, gastrointestinal and bladder function, sexual potency, and vision can all be impaired by autonomic neuropathy damage.

Autonomic neuropathy causes a wide spectrum of nonspecific symptoms ranging from constipation and diarrhea to dizziness and excessive perspiration (see the following table). Unfortunately, these are also common signs of a number of medical conditions, which makes autonomic neuropathy particularly difficult to detect without regular screening. Often, a diagnosis isn't made until organ damage has occurred.

▼ AUTONOMIC NEUROPATHY

Symptoms	Possible Complications
Cardiovascular System	
Dizziness	Orthostatic hypotension
Drop in blood pressure	Silent heart attack
No variation in heart rate	
Elevated resting heart rate	
Shortness of breath	
Perspiration	
Digestive System	
Constipation	Gastroparesis
Diarrhea	
Bloating and nausea	
Premature feeling of fullness	
Genitourinary	
Urinary tract infections	Neurogenic bladder
Urinary incontinence	Nephropathy (kidney damage)
Vaginal dryness	Impotence
Inability to maintain erection	
Decreased or increased urination	
Sudomotor System	
Increased perspiration (trunk and face)	Skin rashes and infection
Decreased perspiration (extremities)	
Dry, thick skin on hands and feet	
Vision	
Small pupils	Impaired night vision
No pupil response to light/dark	

Cardiovascular Autonomic Neuropathy (CAN)

Cardiovascular autonomic neuropathy is a disorder that begins silently. It does not produce symptoms of chest pain or discomfort (angina), and often remains undetected until serious myocardial infarction (death of a portion of the heart muscle due to lack of oxygen) has occurred. As a result, these "silent heart attacks" often pass without proper medical attention.

If you experience any unexplained shortness of breath, weakness and fatigue, and/or excessive perspiration—all possible symptoms of silent heart attack—report these experiences to your doctor. The mortality rate of CAN is up to 50 percent within five years once symptoms appear, so prevention and proper treatment is essential.

QUESTION

I get dizzy when I stand suddenly, and my doctor said it could be neuropathy. Isn't that a foot condition?
Your doctor is talking about autonomic neuropathy. Cardiovascular autonomic neuropathy can trigger a sudden drop in blood pressure known as orthostatic (postural) hypotension. When you stand up, blood vessel and nerve damage prevent your blood pressure from rising quickly enough to compensate for the change in position, and so dizziness, vision problems, and lightheadedness result.

Patients with CAN have little variation in their heart rate, which typically remains continuously elevated both at rest and under stress (i.e., after exercise). Heart rate variability (HRV) testing is used to diagnose the condition. HRV testing involves assessing the heart rate with an electrocardiograph (ECG) during several activities: deep breathing, a postural test (i.e., lying down, rising, and standing), and a Valsalva maneuver. A Valsalva maneuver is performed by bearing down or forcefully breathing out through the mouth with the nose closed. In patients without CAN, the heart rate should slow during this maneuver. If heart rate remains consistent (i.e., does not slow or speeds up) during all three of these activities, CAN is suspected.

Autonomic neuropathy can also cause hypoglycemic unawareness, a potentially serious inability to detect the physical symptoms of a low blood glucose episode.

Cognitive Impairment

People with diabetes may experience memory problems and cognitive impairment. It isn't completely clear, however, whether these problems are a result of the physical processes, the social and psychological toll of the disease, or a combination of the two. There is some evidence that impaired glucose tolerance, a precursor to type 2 diabetes, can cause memory loss and atrophy of the hippocampus (the part of the brain responsible for learning and memory). Recurrent hypoglycemia is also associated with memory loss and worse cognitive function.

Research also shows us that, over time, uncontrolled blood sugar can cause people to have problems with memory and clear thinking, even without a major event such as a stroke. The Action to Control Cardiovascular Risk in Diabetes-Memory in Diabetes (ACCORD-MIND) trial found that among adults with type 2 diabetes, higher A1C levels were associated with lower scores on four different tests of cognitive ability. Further research is necessary to determine the correlation between diabetes and cognitive impairment.

Teeth and Gums

When your diabetes is not well controlled and your body isn't using glucose properly, the extra sugar not only builds up in your blood, but also in your saliva. This makes for a rich breeding ground for bacteria in your mouth, and contributes to tooth and gum disease.

According to the CDC, an estimated one-third of people with diabetes have severe periodontal (gum) disease. And the link between chronic high blood sugar and gum disease is clear. Adults age forty-five and older with an A1C higher than 9 percent are almost three times more likely to develop severe periodontal disease than those without diabetes. That risk is even higher for those who smoke.

Along with good blood sugar control, the best way to keep your mouth healthy and disease free is through good oral care habits. Brush and floss your teeth in the morning, before bed, and after each meal. Use an antiseptic mouthwash after each brushing to eliminate remaining bacteria. And visit your dentist every six months for regular cleanings.

Your Muscles and Bones

In addition to peripheral neuropathy, there are several other complications of diabetes that may affect the musculoskeletal system and the extremities.

Frozen Shoulder

Frozen shoulder, or adhesive capsulitis, is a disorder of the connective tissue that limits the normal range of motion of the shoulder. In diabetes patients, frozen shoulder is thought to be caused by changes to the collagen in the shoulder joint as a result of long-term hyperglycemia. It usually happens in one shoulder only, although it can occur in both. Physical therapy focused on improving range of motion, along with anti-inflammatory medications, are usually the first line of treatment for frozen shoulder. Cortisone injections are sometimes used in treating frozen shoulder, but because of cortisone's propensity to raise blood glucose levels this may not be a preferred treatment.

ALERT

Conditions involving inflammation of the tendons or joints are sometimes treated with nonsteroidal anti-inflammatory medications (NSAIDs), such as ibuprofen or naproxen. However, NSAIDs should be prescribed with care in patients with kidney disease and/or cardiovascular disease, as they have the potential to worsen these conditions.

Dupuytren's Contracture

Another condition that limits range of motion is Dupuytren's contracture. This condition causes the fibrous tissue under the skin of the hand, usually starting on the palm but also extending to the fingers, to thicken and contract or bend inward. The first signs are usually tender nodules felt on the palm. Over time, the fingers are permanently moved. Dupuytren's contracture can be treated with surgery and/or physical therapy.

Stenosing Tenosynovitis, or Trigger Finger

As its common name—trigger finger—suggests, the condition is characterized by a "locking" of the index finger, accompanied by pain and stiffness. The tendon in the finger becomes inflamed and the tendon sheath, or covering, is damaged. Flexing the finger becomes increasingly difficult, and eventually the finger may lock up in a "trigger pull" position. Again, anti-inflammatories and physical therapy may be prescribed. In some cases, surgery may be required to correct the condition.

Carpal Tunnel Syndrome

Often confused with or mistaken for peripheral neuropathy, carpal tunnel syndrome involves nerve entrapment rather than nerve damage. The medial nerve (a nerve that runs through the wrist) becomes compressed, or entrapped, in the ligaments that surround it (the carpal tunnel). This can be caused by repetitive stress (such as that caused by typing at a keyboard or playing guitar), and is exacerbated by diabetes because high blood glucose can cause changes to the collagen in the ligaments, making entrapment more likely.

The result is tingling, "pins and needles," and burning sensations similar to what you might feel in PN. In fact, your doctor may refer to it as a compression neuropathy because it causes these symptoms. The difference is that carpal tunnel usually affects just the first three fingers of the hand (thumb, index, and middle fingers), while PN involves the entire hand.

QUESTION

What is stiff-hand syndrome, and how can I treat it?
Stiff-hand syndrome (digital sclerosis) is caused by a buildup of collagen under the skin. It generally doesn't cause pain, but it can affect your flexibility. A physical therapist can recommend hand-stretching exercises to relieve the stiffness. Another treatment option is paraffin wax, but it should only be applied by a professional because of the risk of burns.

Carpal tunnel syndrome is treated with wrist splints and sometimes corticosteroid injections. In some cases, surgery may be required to relieve pressure on the medial nerve.

Vision Problems

The longer you have had diabetes, the greater your risk for visual complications from the disease. Many people with type 2 diabetes will experience some degree of retinopathy in their lifetime. The good news is that early diagnosis and treatment with laser surgery can prevent serious vision loss in the majority of cases.

Retinopathy

According to the ADA, diabetic retinopathy is the primary cause of new-onset blindness for adults between ages twenty and seventy-four. Retinopathy is caused by blockage and/or leaking of the blood vessels that feed the retina of the eye. Swelling of the macula, which is part of the retina, is called macular edema, a possible complication that can cause blurred vision. Often, symptoms of retinopathy are not noticed until they reach an advanced, or proliferative, stage.

Laser treatment is usually recommended for treating advanced diabetic retinopathy. Depending on the progression of the disease, lasers may be used to either seal leaky blood vessels or completely destroy abnormal vessels.

A vitrectomy, a surgical procedure that replaces the vitreous fluid of the eye with a clear saline solution, may also be performed if blood vessels have hemorrhaged significantly into the vitreous. Both laser treatment and vitrectomy are outpatient procedures performed by an ophthalmologist or eye surgeon.

FACT

If you have diabetes, you are at higher risk for a transient ischemic attack (TIA, or ministroke). A TIA is characterized by symptoms of stroke, but it resolves on its own without treatment. If you think you've had a TIA, call your doctor immediately. It's a warning sign that you are at risk for a full-blown stroke.

Glaucoma

Glaucoma is caused by pressure buildup in the eye that can damage the optic nerve. In cases where the normal drainage patterns of the eye are blocked, the aqueous fluids of the eye build up and put pressure on the optic nerve. A loss of peripheral (side) vision is often the first sign of glaucoma. Depending on the type of glaucoma, you may also experience severe headache. Glaucoma may be treated with special eye drops that lower the pressure level in the eyes. Laser surgery may also be recommended.

Cataracts

People with diabetes tend to develop cataracts at a younger age than the general population. Many people without diabetes also get cataracts, but if you have diabetes, you are twice as likely to develop the condition. Cataracts are characterized by a clouding of the lens of the eye. Symptoms include cloudy or fuzzy vision, double vision, and sensitivity to bright light.

ESSENTIAL

You need a dilated-eye exam at least annually to detect diabetic eye disease early. Other essentials for eye health include kicking the smoking habit and lowering blood pressure, cholesterol, and A1C.

Mild cataracts may not require surgical intervention, unless your vision is significantly reduced. Surgical treatment involves removing the clouded, natural lens and replacing it with a plastic lens calibrated for your vision needs. The prognosis is excellent for anyone undergoing cataract surgery, and the procedure improves vision in well over 90 percent of cases. However, there are some risks for people who also have diabetic retinopathy, as lens replacement can cause a worsening of that condition. Your eye doctor can provide you with information on the risks and benefits of cataract surgery in your specific medical situation.

Hearing Loss

Problems with hearing impairment are twice as common in people with diabetes than in those without. In addition 30 percent of people with prediabetes have some degree of hearing loss. While the relationship between hearing loss and diabetes is not yet determined, researchers think it is caused by damage to nerves and small blood vessels in the ears.

The problem is not just limited to older adults, either. The majority of people with hearing loss in the United States are actually under age sixty-five (although those over sixty-five make up 43 percent of the hearing loss population).

If you find yourself asking others to repeat things often, have trouble hearing high frequency sounds like women's or children's voices, have problems following group conversations, or turn up the volume on music and television to a level others consider too loud, you may be experiencing some hearing loss.

Once again, good diabetes habits that keep blood sugars in a healthy range are the best way to combat hearing problems. If you suspect you might have already developed hearing loss, talk to your doctor. He can arrange to have your hearing tested by a licensed audiologist, who can help determine if a hearing aid is an option for you.

FACT

Sensorineural hearing loss is the most common type of hearing loss for all people, and it is also the type of hearing impairment most associated with diabetes. This type of hearing loss affects your ability to hear very faint sounds, or sounds at a high or low frequency. Sensorineural hearing loss is caused by damage to the inner ear or by damage to the nerves that connect the inner ear to the brain.

Kidney Disease

Your kidneys are two of the hardest working organs in your body. They filter approximately 50 gallons of fluid from the blood that passes through them daily. After the million or so nephrons in each kidney balance electrolytes and filter toxins, 49.5 gallons of fluid are returned to the bloodstream, cleansed, and chemically and hormonally balanced. The remaining half-gallon leaves the body as urine.

Blood vessel damage, hypertension, and insufficiently controlled blood glucose can take a serious toll on renal (or kidney) function, damaging the amazing filtration capacity of the kidneys. As a result, diabetes has become the number one cause of end-stage renal disease (ESRD, or chronic kidney failure), accounting for 44 percent of all U.S. cases.

People with type 2 diabetes are at risk for developing kidney problems, and the risk of developing ESRD increases with the length of time you have had diabetes. This increased risk is probably due to the added stress that high blood pressure and long-term uncontrolled blood glucose place on the kidneys. In fact, uncontrolled hypertension is the second most common cause of kidney failure in America, accounting for 24 percent of the ESRD patient population according to the National Kidney Foundation.

Many people with diabetic kidney disease don't experience any symptoms until the disease has advanced significantly. Signs and symptoms of severe kidney disease include the following:

- Protein (albumin) in the urine
- High blood pressure
- Frequent urination, especially at night
- Leg cramps
- Flank pain
- Puffiness and swelling around the eyes, hands, and feet (edema)
- Excessive itching (pruritis)
- Nausea and vomiting
- Weakness

If your doctor suspects renal impairment, she will run several diagnostic tests to assess your kidney function, including a urine test for microalbumin (trace amounts of protein in the urine). Microalbuminuria is one of the hallmarks of early kidney disease, and at one time was thought to be the beginning of the end of kidney function for people with diabetes. However, recent research shows that with good control of blood glucose, blood pressure, and cholesterol levels, microalbuminuria can be reversed if caught early.

Importance of Good Control

Several large-scale diabetes studies have demonstrated that tight blood sugar control can significantly reduce the risk of nephropathy. The United Kingdom Prospective Diabetes Study (UKPDS) found that people with type

2 diabetes achieved a 35 percent reduction in risk for nephropathy for each lowered percentage point of their A1C levels.

If you develop kidney disease, you may have to watch your protein intake. A registered dietitian can help you to develop a meal plan that is low in dietary protein and compatible with blood sugar control goals. However, studies are still inconclusive on the benefits of low-protein diets in lowering the risk of developing kidney disease. The ADA currently recommends that most adults who have diabetes without known kidney damage should derive approximately 15 to 20 percent of their total dietary calories from protein.

Because diabetic kidney disease often goes hand-in-hand with hypertension, you may be prescribed ACE inhibitors, or other medication, to control your blood pressure and cut the workload of your kidneys as well.

ESSENTIAL

There is no magic pill to reverse kidney failure. Once kidney function diminishes to less than 10 to 15 percent and end-stage renal disease occurs, then hemodialysis, peritoneal dialysis, or kidney transplant are the only treatment options.

Digestive Complications

Gastroparesis, or delayed stomach emptying, literally means stomach weakness. It is another type of autonomic neuropathy. This condition is caused by damage to the vagus nerve, which is responsible for facilitating the passage of food through the digestive system. Gastroparesis is a particular problem for people with diabetes because it can greatly hinder their efforts at blood glucose control. If you can't predict how quickly your food will be digested, your insulin or medication may work too quickly or too slowly.

Symptoms of gastroparesis may include the following:

- Nausea
- Vomiting
- Abdominal bloating
- Weight loss
- Premature feeling of fullness

Dealing with Gastroparesis

Gastroparesis, or slowed digestion that is a form of autonomic neuropathy, can make blood glucose levels hard to handle. People with gastroparesis who take insulin may need to adjust their dosage. Insulin lispro (Humalog, Novo-Log, Apidra) may be recommended since it starts working within minutes and peaks within an hour or two. If you have gastroparesis, your doctor can provide specific recommendations for insulin therapy for your particular situation.

Adjustments to diet are also usually necessary to ease gastroparesis. High-fat and high-fiber foods are discouraged because they slow digestion. Your doctor may recommend eating smaller, more frequent meals, or replacing some meals with liquid-based nutrition.

In cases where vomiting is so extreme that you are having trouble keeping food down altogether, parenteral or jejunostomy (tube) feeding may be required. For cases that are nonresponsive to dietary changes, injections of botulinum toxin (Botox) into the sphincter of the pylorus (the opening connecting the stomach to the small intestine) may be attempted in an effort to relax the opening to allow food to pass through more readily.

FACT

Gastroparesis occurs most frequently in people with type 1 diabetes, and affects an estimated 20 percent of people with the disease. But it is being recognized in a growing number of people with type 2 diabetes. Some studies show that obesity may be a contributing factor to the condition.

Medication may also be prescribed to try to speed up digestion. Commonly prescribed gastroparesis medications include metoclopramide (Reglan, a muscle stimulant), erythromycin (an antibiotic that can speed stomach emptying), and domperidone (Motilium). Domperidone is not approved for use in the United States, but is available in Canada and Europe. U.S. physicians who want to prescribe this drug for gastroparesis patients must complete an Investigational New Drug Application (IND). An IND is a request for FDA authorization to import and administer the drug.

Another medication, cisapride (Propulsid), was withdrawn from the U.S. market by manufacturer Janssen Pharmaceuticals in 2000, but it is still available for qualified patients through a compassionate-use program developed by Janssen and the FDA. Enterra Therapy (Medtronic), a device that uses electrical impulses to stimulate digestion by the stomach, has been successful in treating chronic gastroparesis in some patients for whom drug therapy was not effective. Often described as a pacemaker for the stomach, Enterra is approved as a Humanitarian Use Device (HUD) by the FDA. HUD status means that the device is conditionally cleared by the FDA for use at certain health care centers for treatment of specific rare diseases and conditions.

Skin Conditions

A number of skin conditions can affect people with diabetes. Nerve and small blood vessel damage can make dry skin worse in people with diabetes. Keeping the skin well hydrated is important because any cracks or fissures could easily become infected. In addition to being uncomfortable, the itchiness of dry skin may cause a scratch or abrasion that also poses an infection risk.

Use a humidifier in the home and office, and avoid exposure to harsh detergents and household cleaners that are notorious for drying out skin. If you keep a bottle of hand lotion next to the soap at the kitchen and bathroom sinks, you'll be more likely to remember to use it after each hand washing. In addition, make sure to use mild soap for washing.

"Tougher" areas of the skin, such as the soles of the feet, may benefit from a moisturizing lotion that contains urea (for moisture) and alphahydroxy, or AHA (for sloughing off dead skin). It's a good idea to run any new products past your doctor or CDE (certified diabetes educator) first. Certain areas of your body should be kept dry. Using baby powder in the armpits, between the toes, and other moisture-prone skin-fold areas can help to prevent fungal infections.

People with diabetes frequently develop thickened, shiny areas of skin caused by changes to the collagen fibers. A tendency toward yellow-tinted skin and nails, too, may be triggered by collagen changes (although the cause of this phenomenon isn't completely understood). Other skin conditions that are common in people with diabetes include the following:

- **Acanthosis nigricans:** Dark, thickened patches in the folds of the skin that are common in overweight people with insulin resistance and type 2 diabetes.
- **Bacterial infections:** Staph or strep infections in the skin that may appear as sties, boils, or cellulitis.
- **Fungal infections:** Usually occur in warm, moist areas such as skin folds. Candidiasis (yeast infection), tinea pedis (athlete's foot or ringworm), and tinea cruris (jock itch or ringworm) are all common fungal infections.
- **Diabetic dermopathy:** Brown, scaly rounded patches on the skin that frequently appear on the shins and usually heal on their own.
- **Necrobiosis lipoidica diabeticorum:** Changes in the collagen of the skin that cause large, raised, red, shiny, and sometimes itchy spots. If the spots rupture, they require proper wound care.

Other, less common conditions that may occur in the presence of uncontrolled high blood sugars include bullosis diabeticorum (diabetic blisters) and eruptive xanthomatosis (small, yellow, red-ringed bumps). Both of these conditions usually resolve themselves once blood glucose levels are brought back under control.

Remember, bacterial and fungal infections of the skin require immediate attention and prescription medication to resolve. A dermatologist can diagnose and properly treat any skin conditions you develop, and is yet another essential member of your diabetes care team.

Sleep Disorders

When it comes to getting enough sleep, Americans tend to cheat themselves. Adults need seven to nine hours of quality sleep each night to be at their best; kids and teenagers need even more. Yet according to a U.S. survey conducted by the National Sleep Foundation, 70 percent of adults are regularly getting less than seven hours of sleep per night on weekdays.

Research shows a direct relationship between chronic sleep deprivation and an increased risk of developing type 2 diabetes. In those who already have type 2 diabetes, sleep loss can increase insulin resistance, and can also raise the risk of obstructive sleep apnea and restless leg syndrome, two sleep-stealing disorders. Left untreated, sleep disorders can lead to a vicious cycle of further sleep deficit, worsening both diabetes control and sleep quality.

Sleep Apnea

People with type 2 diabetes are more likely to develop obstructive sleep apnea (OSA). This condition causes periodic and frequent lapses in breathing during sleep. As people with OSA inhale, on occasion the tissues in their throat close off the airways. Obesity can worsen the problem, as fat tissue narrows the airway even further.

During an apnea episode, breathing stops for at least ten seconds and for possibly as long as thirty, until the person suddenly awakens from sleep, catches their breath, and then gradually returns to sleep. This cycle may repeat itself hundreds of times a night, shortening total sleep time and disrupting the quality of sleep.

FACT

Up to 23 percent of people with type 2 diabetes have obstructive sleep apnea. The incidence is even higher for those who are also overweight. In the Look AHEAD trial, a national long-term study of lifestyle factors on weight loss in type 2 diabetes, over 80 percent of enrolled obese patients also suffered from sleep apnea.

Sleep apnea is also associated with high blood pressure. In addition, the sleep disruption that apnea causes can worsen insulin resistance, and therefore make diabetes even more difficult to manage.

Signs of OSA include excessive snoring, waking up from sleep without feeling refreshed, daytime sleepiness, and morning headaches. For short-term relief, a CPAP (continuous positive airway pressure) machine can be effective. The CPAP machine is connected to a mask that is worn over the nose during sleep. As the name suggests, a continuous flow of air helps keep the airway open, which prevents snoring and apnea. Long-term weight loss is critical for overweight people who experience OSA.

Restless Leg Syndrome (RLS)

Can't keep your feet still in bed? Do you experience uncomfortable sensations in your legs and feet in bed that only movement will help? You may have restless leg syndrome, or RLS. People with type 2 diabetes are more likely to develop this nerve-related disorder; and one study found that nearly a third of the enrolled type 2 diabetes patients who previously had no diagnosed sleep disorders, actually had RLS.

The leg and foot discomfort experienced in RLS has been described many ways—burning, pins and needles, skin crawling, aching, shocks, and tingling to name a few. In many cases, these feelings are not unlike peripheral neuropathy symptoms. The difference is that the discomfort is worse at night, and movement of the legs temporarily stops the unpleasant sensation. The need to constantly move one's legs while resting and while sleeping results in poor sleep quality for both the person with RLS and anyone who is sharing their bed.

Applying heat and cold packs to the legs, stretching, regular walking, and massage can all help lessen RLS symptoms. Cutting back on caffeine, nicotine, and alcohol, especially close to bedtime, also helps reduce symptoms because these substances make RLS worse. Iron deficiency can also cause RLS, so your doctor will likely check your iron levels and prescribe a supplement if hemoglobin levels are low. If lifestyle changes or iron supplementation do not help relieve RLS, then drugs that are used to treat Parkinson's disease may be prescribed.

Good Sleep Hygiene

The link between poor sleep and insulin resistance is clear, and it's important for people with type 2 diabetes to give themselves the best circumstances and environments that promote a good night's rest. Some tips to live by:

- **Save the bedroom for sleeping and sex.** Distractions like computers, televisions, and even a book in bed can interfere with a relaxing environment conducive to good sleep—and keep you up later than you should be. If logistics require you to keep these items in your room, plan an early cutoff time for their use and stick to it.

- **Keep things cool.** Keep your bedroom at a comfortable sleeping temperature. Most people prefer, and sleep better in, a cool environment.
- **Quiet down.** It's easier to sleep without the sounds of the outside world intruding. Even something as subtle as a dripping faucet or a ticking clock can be distracting. If outside noise is unavoidable, consider using a white noise machine or ear plugs.
- **Dim the lights.** Light helps to regulate the sleep/wake cycle, so keeping your bedroom dark during sleeping hours is critical. If your job requires shift work or if you face other circumstances that require you to sleep during daylight hours, get light-blocking curtains or shades to keep the room dark.
- **Get comfortable.** If your mattress is seven or more years old, it may be time for a new one. If you are waking up sore, stiff, or not well rested, take a careful look at your mattress and foundation. When buying a replacement, go to a showroom where you can "test drive" each bed to determine the most comfortable mattress option for you.

Your daytime habits can also influence how well you sleep. Make sure your exercise sessions conclude at least three hours earlier than your planned bedtime. It will take your body temperature some time to fall after vigorous exercise, and cooler core body temperatures are associated with better sleep.

Likewise, make sure to eat your meals at least two to three hours before bedtime so that your body can digest the food. And limit fluids close to bedtime to avoid nighttime awakening to visit the bathroom.

If you've followed all these tips and still experience sleep problems, talk to your doctor. She may recommend that you keep a sleep diary—a journal of lifestyle and health habits—so she can pinpoint any trouble spots. Or she may recommend a sleep study to assess the possibility of a sleep disorder. This study involves an overnight stay in a sleep clinic where your breathing, heart rate, and brain activity are measured during sleep. It's important that you get to the bottom of sleep problems to improve both your health and your quality of life.

CHAPTER 13

The Diabetic Foot

What do your feet have to do with diabetes, you ask? A lot. Over time, high blood sugar levels can deaden your nerves and clog up the cardiovascular system, making neuropathy and peripheral vascular disease a real danger to your feet. And with diabetes, your body is slower to heal and is more prone to infection. This means that small blisters and abrasions can quickly turn into serious complications if not treated promptly and properly.

Treat Your Feet Right

The American Podiatric Medical Association (APMA) estimates that the average person walks about 115,000 miles in a lifetime (over four times around the equator, if you're counting). With all that walking, your feet go through a lot of wear and tear. For most people, the pain of a blister or cut is a signal to get off your feet and let them heal. But if you have diabetic neuropathy (nerve damage) in your feet, the pain signal is impaired or gone altogether, and you may not notice an injury until you actually see it.

Daily Foot Check

It only takes a minute to check your feet for signs of abrasions, blisters, or other problems, and it could save you serious medical problems down the road. Make checking your feet a part of your daily routine, either as you get dressed for the day, at shower time, or as you get ready for bed. Before you know it, it will become a healthy habit.

You should give your entire foot the once-over, and check between your toes. If you have flexibility and/or vision problems, and so have trouble seeing everything adequately, ask a family member for help. A flexible, magnified mirror can help you see those hard-to-reach spots.

QUESTION

My fourteen-year-old daughter has diabetes. Do we really have to worry about her feet at such a young age?
While children and teens are less likely than adults to develop foot problems, proper foot care is a good habit to start early. As children grow older, nerve and circulatory impairment will become a bigger risk. In general, people with type 2 diabetes are at greater risk for foot complications.

Blisters, Corns, and Calluses

If you do find a blister, red spot, or cut, clean the surrounding skin and apply a bandage immediately. Do not pop or break a blister, as this will increase your risk of infection. Keep a close eye on the wound and replace the bandage regularly. If the wound starts to get worse, exhibits signs of infection (like pus, redness and warmth, or odor), or doesn't look as if it is healing within a day or so, call your doctor immediately for further instruction.

Keep your feet moisturized to avoid skin fissures or cracks caused by dryness. Do not apply lotion between the toes, as it can breed fungal growth or infection. Instead, sprinkle baby or talcum powder to keep these areas dry. Peripheral neuropathy can cause a 10 percent decrease in skin moisture in the feet, so if you have any degree of PN, take extra care to use skin cream regularly.

If you develop corns or calluses, you're better off letting your podiatrist treat them. If you have PN, do not try to remove corns or calluses with cutting implements or chemical treatments on your own. Use a pumice stone only with your doctor's approval.

Clipping Correctly

To prevent ingrown toenails, clip each nail straight across. And to avoid an accidental slice into your skin, don't cut too close to the skin line. You can smooth out any sharp corners with an emery board. Thick or discolored toenails should be checked out by your podiatrist, as they could be a sign of a fungal infection. If you have mobility problems and have difficulty reaching your feet, get assistance. You can also ask your podiatrist to clip your toenails during your next visit.

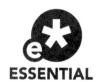

ESSENTIAL

If you must soak in a tub or footbath, only use lukewarm water and make it brief. If you have neuropathy, you could unknowingly burn yourself. When you're done, dry your feet thoroughly with a towel, paying special attention to between your toes. Soaking is never recommended if you have an ulcer or foot wound.

The Right Equipment

Keeping your feet in good condition means proper protection against the elements. The only time you should really go barefoot is in bed and in the shower. Make sure your shoes and socks are appropriate for your needs. An extra investment may be required, but the comfort and reduced risk of complications are well worth the added expense.

Shoes Off the Rack

You have several options for shoes, ranging from regular, off-the-rack footwear to custom-made prescription shoes. If you don't have any diagnosed podiatric conditions, you can probably fulfill your footwear needs at a regular shoe store. However, listed here are some sensible shoe tips you should follow to keep your feet safe:

- **Stay grounded.** High heels are not good for your feet and can cause blisters.
- **On your toes.** Open-toed shoes also present a hazard, as they leave a good portion of your foot exposed. For the best protection, skip the sandals and stay safe.
- **Get fit.** If at all possible, have a trained salesperson check the fit of your shoes in the store. If they don't fit in the store, don't count on them to "stretch" when you get home.
- **Wiggle room.** Properly fitting shoes should leave room for your toes to move freely, and be wide and long enough for a firm yet comfortable fit.
- **Breathing room.** Leather or canvas uppers are your best bet for shoes that allow your feet to breathe, not sweat.
- **Test drive.** Always wear new shoes around the house for short periods in order to break them in and prevent blisters and abrasions. If you get them home and realize they just don't feel right, return them for a better-fitting pair.

ALERT

If you visit the beach, first invest in a pair of hard-soled aqua socks or surf shoes. The sand can be full of hidden hazards like broken glass and sharp seashells, and on a hot day, the possibility of burning your feet is a real danger. Never go without foot protection in the water either.

Shoes by Prescription

If you have existing foot problems, you'll probably need footwear that is a little more customized. Depth shoes are special therapeutic footwear that have extra room for the toes and for any orthotic inserts. If you have foot problems like hammertoes or bunions, depth shoes may be appropriate for you.

Orthotics are prescription devices that are inserted into shoes to relieve pressure and provide extra cushion and support. To produce a custom fit, your podiatrist may take special casts of your feet. Some newer orthotics production technology uses a sensor mat that you walk on to provide a computer-generated view of what portions of your feet bear the greatest load. Special software then designs the specifications for orthotics made to order. Your podiatrist or a specialist called an orthotist or pedorthist (a person trained in the design, fabrication, and fit of orthotic inserts) can help fit you for orthotics.

Health insurance frequently covers the cost of prescription footwear or devices, so check with your carrier. Medicare (Part B) covers 80 percent of the cost of depth-inlay shoes, custom-molded shoes, and shoe inserts for people with diabetes whose doctors certify that they meet clinical qualifications. Your podiatrist can tell you more about your coverage.

ESSENTIAL

Comfort should be a prerequisite for any new pair of shoes you purchase. However, it's still a good idea to break them in gradually to avoid blisters. Wear them around the house for a short period daily for about a week until they start to feel "lived in." Never bring brand-new shoes on vacation as your only footwear option.

Custom-molded shoes may be required for some people with diabetes-related foot deformities such as cases of Charcot foot. Again, these customized shoes are obtained through a podiatrist or orthotist who performs a special casting to fit the shoes properly.

Sock Sense

Even the best-fitting shoes won't do much good if you're wearing thread-bare or hole-riddled socks. Lay a good foundation on your feet with thick, well-cushioned socks that are seamless (to prevent any friction blisters) and wick moisture away from the foot. Cotton, cotton-polyester, or acrylic blends are all good sock material choices. Some newer treated fabrics and blends are now out on the market, such as Teflon and antimicrobial fibers, and designed to prevent blisters and infection. Because socks are a relatively small investment, it's a good idea to try out a variety until you find a type that suits you in style and comfort.

Tight and restrictive elastic bands (such as those on hosiery) can cut off circulation, but some degree of compression built into the sock construction can be supportive and help to protect against deep-vein thrombosis. Other people, particularly those with edema (swollen feet), may do better with a loose-fitting sock. Your podiatrist can advise you on what's right for your particular needs.

Monofilament Test

Peripheral neuropathy (PN), or nerve damage of the extremities, is one of the most common complications of diabetes (60 percent of all people with the disease develop it at some point). Symptoms of PN include burning, tingling, numbness, a prickly sensation (like "pins and needles"), and muscle weakness. Neuropathy is the result of chronically high blood sugars, so the best way to prevent it is to maintain good glucose control.

To check for neuropathy, your doctor should perform a monofilament test—a measure of the sensation in your feet—at least annually. In this simple yet sensitive evaluation, the doctor uses the monofilament, which is a piece of plastic fiber resembling fishing line, to touch various parts of the sole of your foot, and then assesses your ability to feel it at varying pressure. This assessment is sometimes called the 10-gram monofilament test because the fiber is calibrated to bend to 10 grams of pressure. People with diabetes can get a free monofilament testing kit from the Lower Extremity Amputation Prevention (LEAP) program at *www.hrsa.gov/leap*.

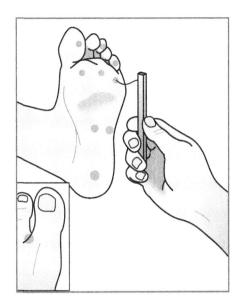

The monofilament test for peripheral neuropathy.

Your doctor may also use a tuning fork on the bottoms of your feet to see if you can sense the vibration. Nerve-conduction studies or velocity tests, which use electrodes to stimulate nerves and then measure the resulting impulses, are a less frequently used but more sophisticated method of diagnosing some neuropathies. Electromyography (EMG), which uses thin needles inserted into the muscles to measure electrical impulses, may also be performed. These latter two tests can be painful, and will likely not be ordered unless there is some question about the diagnosis.

When to See a Podiatrist

For people with neuropathy, the ADA recommends a thorough foot exam at least annually and a visual inspection of the feet at each regular physician's appointment. Your regular doctor may perform these tests, or she may refer you to a podiatrist. A doctor of podiatric medicine (DPM) is a medical doctor with specialized training in the physiology and medical care of the foot and ankle. Podiatrists are licensed in all fifty states.

If you have diagnosed structural, nerve, or skin problems with your feet, a podiatrist should be on your diabetes care team, and you should see him every three to six months. Foot ulcers, in particular, require specialized wound care to avoid infection and possible amputation.

In addition to the regular tests for neuropathy described previously, a podiatrist will assess the pulse of the foot and ankle (pedal pulse) and the temperature of your feet to screen for circulatory problems. Blood pressure readings of both the ankle and the arm are also performed with a cuff, and ultrasound or Doppler may be used to check blood flow.

ALERT

Add diabetic foot problems to the long list of negative health effects from smoking. Smoking tobacco constricts your blood vessels, which can make circulatory problems worse and restrict blood flow to your feet.

Charcot Foot or Joint

Charcot foot or joint, also called neuropathic arthropathy, is a podiatric condition that occurs in a small percentage of people who suffer from diabetic peripheral neuropathy. This condition is caused by a breakdown of the joints and bones that goes unnoticed because of nerve damage and results in deformities of the bones of the feet. A podiatrist or an orthopedist usually treats the condition.

Typical signs of Charcot foot include extreme swelling, warmth of the skin, and redness. Since these are also signs of infection, cellulitis, or deep-vein thrombosis, x-ray examination is needed to confirm the diagnosis.

The Healing Process

In order to heal properly, a Charcot foot must be immobilized in a contact cast, which is replaced periodically in order to inspect the foot. This foot-to-upper-leg cast cushions and protects the foot, and in many cases you may be able to walk on it with the help of crutches or a cane. However, some patients may be instructed to stay off their feet completely.

The cast may need to stay on as long as six months while the foot heals; after it is removed, a leg brace may be required. Frequently, pressure ulcers form as a result of the foot deformity and consequent redistribution of weight. As new bone forms, deformities usually develop that will require custom-molded footwear to accommodate them after the cast is removed. Reconstructive surgery may be required in extreme cases where ulcers become a recurring problem. Physical therapy can also help you regain motion and learn adaptive exercise techniques.

FACT

Diabetes is the leading cause of lower-extremity amputation in the United States, accounting for over 60 percent of nontraumatic limb amputation in America. The good news is at least half of all amputations can be prevented with early intervention and proper foot and skin care.

Diabetic Foot Ulcers

If you've ever had a shot of Novocain at the dentist, you know how difficult it can be to talk or eat immediately afterward—kind of like knitting with boxing gloves on. People who have lost the sensation in their feet have a similar experience. Neuropathy often causes an unnatural and awkward stride, which puts repeated pressure on the same spot of your foot. Over time, this area will form calluses and may eventually develop into a pressure ulcer. Poor circulation in your legs and feet may also cause other diabetic foot ulcers. Often, ulcers become infected and then serious problems can set in. Beyond practicing good foot care, the best thing you can do to prevent limb-threatening complications from ulcers is to detect them early and treat them properly.

How Ulcers Happen

Most ulcers form on the bottom of the foot, although shoes that don't fit well can cause sores and subsequent ulcers on the top of the foot or the ankle. Usually ulcers start as a callus, small sore, abrasion, or blister that would be "no big deal" for someone without diabetes. However, chronic high blood sugar levels, poor circulation, and nerve damage are a recipe for ulceration in people with diabetes.

There are two categories of foot ulcers: vascular and neuropathic (or "pressure"). The former is caused by peripheral vascular disease (PVD)—blockages of the arteries that carry blood to the feet. The latter is the result of the loss of sensation that accompanies peripheral neuropathy (PN). People who have PN may put increased pressure on the same area of their foot repeatedly, which results in callusing at first, and eventually in ulceration. Ulcers caused by PVD are usually painful, while those caused by PN are usually not.

ESSENTIAL

Keep those feet moving to promote good circulation and ward off vascular ulcers. Exercise (low-impact if you have foot problems), avoid sitting with your legs crossed for more than a few minutes at a time, and periodically stretch your legs and toes. Raising your feet slightly when you're at rest can also help blood flow to the feet.

Treatment

Infection is the primary risk with foot ulcers, so proper wound care is essential. Ulcers should remain moist and covered in a breathable dressing at all times (except when changing bandages). Oxygen is essential to the healing process. Oral antibiotic medication may also be prescribed if infection is present. If you have a pressure ulcer, your podiatrist (or orthopedic or plastic surgeon) may perform debridement—removal of callused, dead skin.

Ulcers that are the result of PVD may show up on the lower leg as well as on the foot. The toes are also a common location for ulcers, and if circulation is poor enough, tissue necrosis (tissue death) or gangrene may be evident in the surrounding blackened skin. These patients may need an arterial bypass to restore blood flow to their feet and legs and to prevent amputation.

Osteomyelitis, or bone infection, may occur if infection in the ulcer spreads deeply enough. This condition is usually diagnosed with a bone scan or magnetic resonance imaging (MRI) and treated with intravenous antibiotic therapy.

FACT

According to the National Institutes of Health (NIH), an estimated 15 percent of people with diabetes develop a foot ulcer at some point. Prompt and proper care is the best way to avoid ulcers and their related complications.

Your doctor may also prescribe one of several new "human-based" products, such as Apligraf (Organogenesis) and Dermagraft (Advanced BioHealing). Apligraf and Dermagraft are bioengineered tissues containing skin cells and proteins that promote healing and new skin growth. Both can be useful to treat ulcers that haven't healed with conventional methods.

Another promising wound therapy is hyperbaric oxygen treatment (HBOT), a method which speeds wound healing by delivering 100 percent oxygen therapy to the affected area in a pressurized chamber. The hyperbaric chamber is either a small extremity chamber that your leg or foot fits into, called a topical treatment, or a full-body chamber that you lie in. Due to limited availability and high cost, HBOT is usually not a first-line treatment for diabetic foot wounds.

Your best protection against diabetes-related foot problems is maintaining good blood glucose control. It is also essential for you to keep your heart and circulatory system healthy by watching what you eat, maintaining cholesterol and blood pressure levels within normal limits, and staying active.

CHAPTER 14

Tests, Tests, and More Tests

The average person with diabetes racks up $11,744 in medical care annually. Although the price tag sounds high, the toll of uncontrolled blood sugar levels and associated complications in the United States is much higher—an estimated $116 billion in direct medical costs each year. Think of all the prescriptions, lab work, and doctor's visits as preventive maintenance. Like spending money to restore a vintage car, your investment will pay big dividends in smooth operation and enjoyment later.

The A1C Test

In addition to your home blood sugar monitoring routine, covered elsewhere in this book, you'll be donating quite a bit of blood to the testing cause at your doctor's office or lab. One of the most important of these tests is the glycosylated hemoglobin test (also called a glycated hemoglobin test, GHB, or HbA1c). The A1C assesses your long-term, three-month glucose average.

Glycosylated hemoglobin is a substance produced when excess glucose attaches itself to hemoglobin (a substance in red blood cells). The higher your percentage of glycated hemoglobin, the higher your blood glucose levels were over the past ninety-day period. The ADA recommends that an A1C be performed at least twice annually, and up to four times a year for individuals who are undergoing adjustments to treatment or failing to meet treatment goals. Patients who use insulin to control their type 2 diabetes should have the test performed quarterly as well. Pregnant patients with pre-existing diabetes will probably have more frequent A1C tests at four- to six-week intervals.

Long-Term Control

A1C levels are the best measure of how you're doing in the long term. While home monitoring offers you a single snapshot of where your blood sugar is at a particular point in time, an A1C test is like a surveillance camera running for three months, day and night, giving you an overview of your average blood glucose levels.

FACT

In 2007, the International Federation of Clinical Chemistry and Laboratory Medicine (IFCC) adopted a new reference value for the A1C test called eAG (estimated average glucose), which translates the A1C to an average daily blood sugar value. For example, an A1C of 7 has an eAG of 154 mg/dl. The ADA recommends that laboratories processing A1C tests also provide an eAG value to health care providers.

The A1C not only looks back at the past three months, but also provides a glimpse into your future risk of complications. The United Kingdom

Prospective Diabetes Study (UKPDS), a landmark clinical study, found that participants with type 2 diabetes who kept their A1C values below 7 percent had a 25 percent reduction in the incidence of microvascular complications such as retinopathy, nephropathy, and neuropathy. And for every percentage point decrease in A1C achieved, there was a 35 percent reduction in the risk of these eye, kidney, and nervous system complications.

ALERT

Certain conditions and substances can affect the results of an A1C test. Vitamins C and E, opiates, and salicylates like aspirin can influence results of some A1C tests, as can iron-deficiency anemia and chronic alcoholism.

Determining Your Target Goal

People without diabetes have an A1C of around 5 percent. It is possible for people with well-controlled diabetes to achieve A1C levels in a range very close to normal. The American Association of Clinical Endocrinologists (AACE) recommends that individuals with diabetes try to achieve a target A1C of 6.5 percent or less to minimize the risk of long-term complications. The American Diabetes Association (ADA) suggests an A1C goal of less than 7 percent for the general diabetes population, although it acknowledges that "selected individual patients" can strive for a goal of 6 percent or lower. However, the ADA also suggests that older patients, small children, and those with certain health conditions may have higher goals. The bottom line is that everyone is different and you should work with your health care provider to find the A1C target that is right for you.

ALERT

If severe hypoglycemia is a problem for you, your doctor may recommend slightly higher A1C goals. Hypoglycemic unawareness, blood sugar lows that occur without symptoms, may also be an indication that a higher A1C target is warranted. Talk with your doctor about what's right for you.

The UKPDS found that the closer to normal you can bring your A1C, the lower your risk for microvascular complications. But don't be discouraged if your initial A1C tests are higher. Target A1C levels are as individual as diabetes itself. Your doctor will look at your medical history, age, lifestyle, and other factors, and will work with you to define a custom target goal specific to your needs. It can take some time to get your A1C where you want it. In the UKPDS, the average A1C at time of type 2 diagnosis was 9.3 percent, which leaves a lot of room for improvement.

Other Glucose Tests

Your provider may do a random blood glucose test to check the accuracy of your self-monitoring and/or your home meter. She may also test your glucose levels if she is adjusting your medication or treatment routine. Results are provided in plasma glucose values.

The Fructosamine Test

This is another test that measures your blood sugar over a period of time (two to three weeks, as opposed to the eight to twelve weeks measured by the A1C test). The fructosamine test is a measurement of glycated serum proteins, and may be used as a companion to A1C when you want to find out how blood glucose control has responded to treatment changes in a shorter time period. It may also be used along with an A1C during pregnancy when treatment needs may change rapidly. And it is sometimes recommended for people with certain blood disorders for which the A1C is not a reliable marker. However, for most people, the fructosamine test should not be thought of as a replacement for daily blood sugar monitoring or A1C tests.

Urine Glucose Tests

Available as reagent "dipstick" tests, urinary glucose tests were once the standard method of measuring glucose levels at home for people with diabetes. With the advent of accurate home monitoring systems, urine glucose tests are now usually relegated to the purpose of infrequent screening. These tests have several drawbacks. First, they are time-delayed—they can't tell you what your blood glucose level is right now, but only several hours later after glucose has filtered into the urine and urine has collected in the bladder and is ready to leave the body. They are also not highly sensitive or specific; a negative urine test can ensure only that your blood glucose levels are below 180 mg/dl (10.0 mmol/l), well above a "controlled" range for most people. And unlike a blood glucose monitor, they cannot detect blood glucose lows at all.

Blood testing is the gold standard for SMBG (self-monitoring of blood glucose levels). However, urine glucose test strips are sometimes used by patients who simply cannot afford blood-monitoring supplies. They may also be used by patients who can't or won't blood-test due to discomfort or other reasons. If you're having financial difficulties, talk to your health care provider about patient assistance programs that can provide blood glucose testing supplies free of charge.

What about Insulin Tests?

There are several ways of testing glucose levels, but what about insulin testing? There is a way to test insulin—the insulin serum test, which measures the amount of insulin in the bloodstream. However, given its expense and lack of clinical usefulness, it is rarely used in diabetes diagnosis and assessment. Insulin has a short half-life and is significantly cleared from the body before it even reaches the general circulation. In addition, the test does not differentiate between injected and endogenous (or self-produced) insulin. Instead of testing insulin, assessing levels of c-peptide, a more accurate predictor of beta cell function, is more common.

Lipid Profile

Because cardiovascular disease is the leading cause of death among people with diabetes, the ADA recommends an annual fasting lipid panel as part of regular preventive diabetes care. If you are working with your physician to control lipid levels through medication or diet, testing may be done more often.

A fasting lipid profile is a blood test that assesses your risk for developing cardiovascular complications by measuring levels of total cholesterol, high-density lipoprotein (HDL or "good") cholesterol, triglycerides, and low-density lipoprotein (LDL or "bad") cholesterol. It is also used to diagnose dyslipidemia, a condition characterized by unhealthy blood lipid, or fat, profiles. This includes the high triglyceride and low HDL cholesterol levels that are common in type 2 diabetes and increase the overall risk of heart disease.

▼ CHOLESTEROL LEVELS RECOMMENDED FOR GENERAL DIABETES POPULATION

	NCEP* Guidelines	ADA and AACE Guidelines
Total cholesterol	<200 mg/dl	N/A
HDL	>40 mg/dl	>40 mg/dl (men) and >50 mg/dl (women)
LDL	<100 mg/dl	<100 mg/dl
Triglycerides	<150 mg/dl	<150 mg/dl

*The National Cholesterol Education Program

People with diabetes and existing cardiovascular disease may have more stringent cholesterol goals. Talk to your health care provider about the cholesterol targets that are right for you. Medical history, gender, age, ethnicity, and even geographic region of origin can affect cholesterol levels. Triglyceride levels can be raised by kidney and liver disease and alcoholism. High serum cholesterol levels can be triggered by poor dietary habits, pancreatitis, hypothyroidism, genetic lipid disorders, and certain kidney and liver diseases. High LDL levels reflect an increased risk of coronary artery disease.

More Cardiovascular Tests

The ADA suggests that primary-care physicians assess their patients' heart disease risk factors annually and prescribe cardiac testing accordingly. Cardiac testing may include an electrocardiogram (ECG), a stress test, or an echocardiogram.

Electrocardiogram (ECG, or EKG)

An ECG measures the electrical impulses put out by the heart and creates a visual representation, or tracing, of them. The test is used to check for irregularities in heart rhythm or rate and to detect signs of coronary artery disease or heart damage.

ESSENTIAL

Since an electrocardiogram is fairly inexpensive and noninvasive, your physician may perform it on an annual basis or even more frequently, especially if you have a history of heart disease or other additional risk factors besides your diabetes.

For a resting ECG, you will be asked to lie flat on a table while sensor patches (leads) are attached to ten various points on the body. The sensors are attached to wires that transfer your heart's electrical impulses into the ECG unit where a tracing is generated. The test is very brief, taking only about five to ten minutes from start to finish. Your physician will then review the tracing for abnormalities that may indicate an artery blockage or other heart problems.

Exercise Stress Test

As the name implies, an exercise stress test evaluates how your heart and cardiovascular system perform under the pressure of exercise. Your heart is again monitored with ECG leads and a blood pressure cuff. A pulse oximeter (a small, painless clamp that uses light to measure the level of oxygen in your bloodstream) is attached to a finger or other site with sufficient blood flow. Baseline levels of your heart function are taken at rest before the stress test begins.

A stress test is usually performed on a treadmill or stationary bicycle. The level of exertion, or stress, is increased periodically until the patient reaches a specific heart rate. Each time the stress increases, vital signs are measured. The test will be stopped if chest pain, dangerously high blood pressure, or other danger signs develop. The whole procedure typically takes about fifteen to twenty minutes, and your heart will continue to be monitored after the exercise portion ends until vital signs return to baseline levels.

Echoes and Scans

Your primary-care provider may also recommend other tests that assess cardiac function and structure, including nuclear perfusion and echocardiography. The nuclear perfusion test, sometimes called a thallium scan or a Cardiolite scan, uses a trace amount of radioactive material injected into the bloodstream. The radioactive material is absorbed by cardiac muscle and allows better visualization of the heart structures using a special camera. Poor absorption is associated with inadequate blood flow (perfusion) and may indicate that the arteries leading to that portion of the heart are diseased. A Cardiolite scan also allows the physician to visualize coronary arterial disease (CAD) and areas of tissue death signifying a previous myocardial infarction, or heart attack. Echocardiography, or "echo," uses ultrasound to see the heart. A small wand, called a transducer, is passed over the chest and sound waves emitted by the transducer bounce off the structures of the heart. The resulting image is displayed on a video screen. Blood flow is also visible.

Kidney Function Tests

Diabetes is the leading cause of chronic kidney failure, or end-stage renal disease (ESRD). Uncontrolled high glucose levels can damage the nephrons—the filtering units of the kidney that remove excess fluids and waste products from the bloodstream. Regular screening for early signs of kidney problems is an essential part of diabetes care.

Testing for Protein

Healthy kidneys should filter and absorb proteins instead of excreting them into the urine. A microalbumin test detects the presence of the protein albumin in the urine—a sign of kidney disease or damage. Chemical reagent test strips (dipsticks) may be used to screen for protein. They are quick and easy, requiring only a small urine sample and a few minutes for testing. However, they should be performed in conjunction with a urine creatinine test, described later in this chapter, to be clinically accurate in assessing kidney function.

FACT

In a twenty-four-hour urine collection, up to 150 milligrams of protein excreted in a twenty-four-hour period is considered normal. Moderate levels of protein (0.5 to 4.0 g/24 hours) are often present in renal disease as a complication of diabetes. High levels (over 4.0 g/24 hours) occur in nephrotic syndrome. Because this test is cumbersome, it is not prescribed often.

The preferred test for microalbuminuria screening is a random spot test taken at your doctor's office or a lab that analyzes both albumin and creatinine levels, called the albumin-to-creatinine ratio. Values of 30 to 299 milligrams signal microalbuminuria, one of the earliest signs of diabetic nephropathy (kidney disease). Levels of 300 milligrams or more indicate macroalbuminuria, which is a hallmark of early end-stage renal disease (ESRD). However, the diagnosis of microalbuminuria or macroalbuminuria should be confirmed in two of three random specimens taken within a three- to six-month time frame.

ALERT

If microalbumin is present on several consecutive tests, it usually indicates diabetic nephropathy, or kidney disease due to diabetes. Bladder infection and/or nephritis, and menstruation can also cause an elevated microalbumin level, as can high blood pressure and periods of hyperglycemia.

Screening for microalbuminuria should be performed annually. Current ADA guidelines for people with type 2 diabetes recommend that screening starts at diagnosis and take place every year thereafter. It may be performed more often with those patients at high risk for renal disease. If microalbumin is present on a test, a repeat test should be performed to confirm the results.

Serum Creatinine

The ADA recommends that all people with diabetes undergo annual testing of serum (or blood) creatinine levels to assess kidney function. Creatinine is a metabolic by-product of creatine, the acid that supplies energy for muscle contractions. Creatinine is filtered out of the bloodstream by the kidneys. Creatinine blood levels greater than 1.2 mg/dl for women and 1.4 mg/dl for men points to inadequate filtering by the kidneys (renal impairment), although normal creatinine values do vary by age.

Serum creatinine values help your physician calculate your glomerular filtration rate (GFR), or the rate at which your kidneys are filtering waste and fluids from your body. The GFR is also used to stage kidney disease; a GFR of less than 15 indicates kidney failure (stage 5, or end-stage renal failure). A GFR of less than 60 for three months or longer is considered diagnostic of chronic kidney disease. Although "normal" GFR values vary by age, sex, and body type, if your GFR is over 90 and you have no evidence of protein in the urine, then your kidneys are most likely healthy.

FACT

Can't keep your creatinine straight? Just remember that healthy, functioning kidneys will cleanse this waste product from the blood and move it into the urine for disposal—so serum levels should be low and urine levels should be high.

Urine Creatinine Clearance

Creatinine clearance measures the kidney's ability to filter creatinine from the blood. Normal kidneys should filter creatinine, a waste product, into the urine at a constant rate.

Before a creatinine clearance urine test is performed, a blood sample is taken to determine the level of creatinine in the bloodstream (serum creatinine, described earlier). A urine specimen is then analyzed for creatinine output, and the creatinine clearance is computed by comparing the urine creatinine to the original blood creatinine levels. If kidney function is impaired, creatinine levels in the urine will be low. Low creatinine clearance levels may indicate kidney disease (i.e., polycystic kidney disease, glomeru-lonephritis), congestive heart failure, and/or severe dehydration.

Blood Urea Nitrogen (BUN)

Urea is another waste product that is filtered from the blood by the kidneys. Urea is generated in the liver by metabolized protein. Elevated BUN levels on a blood test indicate a slowdown in kidney function. Normal adult BUN levels are between 7 and 20 mg/dl. BUN will rise as kidney function falls. An elevated BUN is also a sign of several other possible conditions, including dehydration, congestive heart failure, excessive protein intake, internal bleeding, and heart attack.

Ketones and Diabetic Ketoacidosis

Ketones are formed when the body can't use insulin to process glucose into fuel and is forced to burn fat for energy. Trace amounts of ketones are not unusual and are usually no cause for alarm, but when accompanied by elevated blood sugars in high enough levels, they can be a sign of diabetic keto-acidosis (DKA), a potentially fatal medical emergency. DKA usually occurs in situations where someone has stopped taking needed insulin injections, is taking an insufficient dose of insulin, or is taking contaminated, expired, or otherwise bad insulin. The physical stress of a flu, cold, or other illness usually increases both blood glucose levels and the need for insulin, and DKA often occurs in these situations.

ESSENTIAL

Consider checking your urine for ketones if your blood glucose levels are 250 mg/dl or higher for two or more consecutive readings. It's a good idea to ask your doctor, before you get ill, if ketone testing should be a part of your "sick-day routine."

If your provider suspects the onset of DKA, she will probably check the level of ketones in your blood. This test may also be performed as part of a routine urinalysis. However, there is also a urine test (frequently used at home) to check for the presence of ketones. The test uses a chemically treated reagent strip (Ketostix) that is dipped in a urine sample to check for the presence of ketones. The strip changes color, and the color is matched to an enclosed chart that indicates the presence and level of ketones in the urine.

Some people with type 2 diabetes, including children and pregnant women, may be advised to keep ketone test strips on hand at home. In situations where your blood sugar is prone to go high—such as when you are ill—monitoring of urinary ketone levels is essential for preventing ketoacidosis. If testing indicates the presence of moderate or high levels of ketones, you should contact your doctor immediately or go to an emergency care facility.

Comprehensive Eye Exam

Diabetes can cause blood vessels in the retina to become damaged or blocked, resulting in vision loss—a condition known as diabetic retinopathy. The National Eye Institute (NEI) estimates that half of all people with diabetes will develop retinopathy at some point in their lifetime. They are also at risk for developing cataracts and glaucoma, which may impair vision.

ALERT

Pregnant women with pre-existing type 2 diabetes (not gestational diabetes) should have a dilated-eye examination during the first trimester of pregnancy to screen for microvascular (blood vessel) problems, with exams through pregnancy and the postpartum period. This is because retinopathy may worsen during pregnancy. The ADA also recommends a preconception eye examination.

Both the ADA and the NEI recommend an annual dilated-eye exam for people with type 2 diabetes. Your first exam should be at or shortly following diagnosis. If you have diagnosed eye disease, you may require more frequent assessment to monitor treatment and disease progression.

In a dilated-eye exam, eyedrops are used to counteract the reflexes that normally trigger the pupil to shrink in bright light. The ophthalmologist or optometrist uses a high-intensity focused light called a slit-lamp to illuminate the eye. Dilation opens up the pupil, allowing the ophthalmologist to view the back, or fundus, of the eye and the blood vessels and optic nerve situated there. The ophthalmologist may also perform an intravenous fluorescein angiography, in which dye is injected into your veins to better visualize the blood vessels in the eye.

An intraocular pressure test, also called a tonometry test, is used to screen for glaucoma. Tonometry is sometimes called a puff test because it may involve blowing a quick puff of air at your eye and measuring the resistance it meets. Another type of pressure test, applanation, uses fluorescein dye to temporarily color the cornea before a tonometer instrument is placed against the eye to measure fluid pressure. Anesthetic drops are used to prevent any discomfort.

Other parts of a comprehensive eye exam may include the following tests:

- **Visual acuity test:** The familiar Snellen eye chart
- **Visual field test:** A test of your peripheral (side) vision
- **Refraction test:** Checks how light reflects, or refracts, off your retina
- **Binocular test:** Assesses your eye teamwork—how well the muscle coordination and control of your eyes work in tandem

If you wear glasses or contact lenses, your exam should also include an evaluation of your current prescription.

CHAPTER 15

Women and Diabetes

Feeling as if you're in a permanent state of PMS—even if you're well past menopause? The hormonal tides of puberty, pregnancy, menstruation, and menopause are each yet another seismic force to contend with as you try to maintain balance and control of your diabetes. Remember that treatment is not a static thing; "adapt, adapt, and adapt" will be your motto as you move through the stages of diabetes care.

At Puberty

The barrage of hormones, social turmoil, fashion crises, and other adolescent dramas that spells puberty can also spell trouble for your teen's (or pre-teen's) diabetes control. Issues of poor self-image and of wanting to fit in with peers by acting and eating as they do may raise blood sugar levels, either through noncompliance with treatment or as a stress response. Hormonal changes, which magnify all of the preceding and can increase the need for insulin, compound the problem.

FACT

Studies show that overweight and obese prepubertal girls have both increased insulin resistance and on average, an earlier onset of menarche (the first menstrual period) than normal weight counterparts. And early menarche has been associated with an increased risk of type 2 diabetes and weight problems later in life.

Many overweight and obese girls at risk for type 2 diabetes are diagnosed with the condition when puberty hits due to this "perfect storm" of hormonal changes. Metformin, along with recommended changes to diet and exercise, is usually the first line treatment for these girls.

At Risk for Eating Disorders

Binge eating, the consumption of large amounts of food and a self-perceived loss of control, can be a troubling problem for girls with type 2 diabetes. The TODAY (Treatment Options for Type 2 Diabetes in Adolescents and Youth) study found that 26 percent of children and teens with type 2 reported regular binge eating. These kids were more likely to be obese, suffer from depression, and have a diminished quality of life.

Binge eating leads to high blood sugars but also worsens existing weight problems. This leads to a vicious cycle of not just increased insulin resistance, but depression, poor self-esteem, and other psychological issues. If you suspect your child may be having difficulties with binge eating, it's important to get help from a qualified mental health-care provider.

Diabetes and Menstruation

If you are a premenopausal woman with diabetes, you may notice a rise in blood glucose levels as your menstrual period draws closer. The rise in estrogen and progesterone levels that occurs toward the end of the cycle (about a week before menstruation) can increase insulin resistance, causing a rise in glucose levels. In other women with diabetes, this hormonal change may actually increase insulin sensitivity, triggering lower blood sugar levels. And in line with the true one-size-fits-none nature of diabetes, some women may experience no changes at all.

Tracking your glucose levels throughout your monthly cycle can help you understand if hormones are having an impact on your diabetes control (yet one more thing to keep in your blood glucose log). Discuss your results with your doctor or diabetes educator. Adjustments in medication, insulin, exercise, and diet may be necessary to bring your glucose levels back to normal during this time.

Pregnancy: Treatment for Two

Having a baby is not a decision to be entered into lightly for anyone. For women with diabetes, the decision may be even more difficult because of the demands placed on their body, the necessity for painstaking control before and during the pregnancy, and the potential for developing or worsening diabetic complications in the process.

Some complications of diabetes, including retinopathy, nephropathy, and neuropathy, can get worse in pregnancy. Your doctor will counsel you about your specific risks as part of preconception planning. Tests that may be ordered during preconception planning include:

- A1C
- Kidney function (serum creatinine, twenty-four-hour urine)
- Comprehensive eye exam
- Cardiovascular screening

Control Before Conception

When it comes to having a successful pregnancy with type 2 diabetes, planning is everything. Achieving good blood sugar control before conception is the best way to ensure a good outcome for both you and your child. The ADA recommends that women who plan on becoming pregnant strive for an A1C level of less than 7 percent.

If you take drugs for hypertension or other diabetic complications, your doctor will discuss your options with you, as many of these drugs are not recommended for pregnancy. Drug therapy that is contraindicated in pregnancy, including oral diabetes medications, will likely have to be stopped and replaced with insulin therapy (which is considered safe in pregnancy). Starting insulin before you try to conceive will give you the chance to become accustomed to the routine and make appropriate dosage adjustments for optimal control.

Ideally, blood glucose will be stabilized at the target goal, or as close as possible to it, for several months before you try to conceive. Adjustments to insulin and other aspects of your treatment will probably have to be made during pregnancy, too, which is why it's important to continue to involve your endocrinologist or diabetes care specialist, as well as your ob-gyn, in your treatment throughout your pregnancy.

FACT

Diabetic retinopathy is one condition that pregnancy may make worse. The ADA recommends that in addition to a dilated-eye exam during preconception planning, women who become pregnant have a comprehensive eye exam in the first trimester and close follow-up with an ophthalmologist throughout pregnancy.

Staying Healthy During Pregnancy

Once you become pregnant, your provider may recommend that you see a perinatologist, an ob-gyn who specializes in high-risk pregnancies. As with any member of your diabetes care team, you should make sure the physician you choose communicates clearly and proactively with you and your other providers, answers your questions to your satisfaction, and encourages you to play an active role in your treatment.

Your insulin needs may go up in pregnancy, as your placenta starts to manufacture hormones that increase your insulin resistance. Frequent glucose checks during this time are critical, and your doctor may also administer A1C testing every four to six weeks instead of the typical three-month interval.

Your Baby and Diabetes

Get your baby's doctor on board early. A neonatologist, a doctor who cares for newborns with special health needs, may be consulted and asked to be in the delivery room at birth in case of any problems. Choosing a pediatrician early is also a good idea.

If you are able to keep your blood sugar well controlled during pregnancy, your baby's risk of complications is reduced dramatically. Tight control in the first trimester in particular is important, because this is the critical time when the fetus's organ systems are developing.

QUESTION

I have had type 2 diabetes for five years, and my doctor just added a diagnosis of PCOS. Are they related?
Just like type 2 diabetes, polycystic ovary syndrome (PCOS) is characterized by insulin resistance. High cholesterol, hypertension, and heart disease are also hallmark characteristics. PCOS triggers an overabundance of androgens (male sex hormones) and too little estrogen, causing cysts to form in the ovaries.

Babies born to mothers with diabetes have a greater chance of being born large for birth weight. This is because the fetus converts extra glucose into body fat in the womb. The condition, called macrosomia, puts newborns at risk for unplanned C-section birth and shoulder dystocia (which results from getting wedged in the birth canal during delivery).

When the hard work of active labor starts to kick into high gear, your insulin needs will drop. This is, after all, the ultimate form of exercise. And just like a strenuous workout, you run the risk of going low. Your glucose levels will be tested regularly, and you may have an IV line or heparin lock inserted to infuse glucose or insulin as needed. Talk to your ob-gyn or peri-natologist well before your due date to discuss the protocol used to prevent hypos in labor.

Because of your medical history, your labor and delivery team will be on the lookout for hypoglycemia. While still in your womb, your baby's pancreas had been programmed to produce enough insulin to counteract your sometimes-heightened blood glucose supply. Once he becomes "disconnected" from the maternal sugar source at delivery, his high insulin levels may drive his blood glucose down, causing hypoglycemia. A heel stick blood test can confirm the diagnosis, and oral glucose or a glucose IV drip for your baby can quickly treat the condition.

Type 2 diabetes does have a strong hereditary link. If a child has one parent with type 2 diabetes, his risk of developing the disease is 3.5 times higher than a child of a parent without diabetes. If both parents have type 2, his risk is six times higher. But the good news is that genetic risk alone is not enough; it usually requires an environmental "trigger"—like a sedentary lifestyle or poor eating habits that lead to weight problems—to cause diabetes. And in many cases, it can be prevented with healthy lifestyle changes.

Breastfeeding

Many women with diabetes question their ability to breastfeed, worrying about either harm to their baby—Is my milk safe? Does it have enough nutrients?—or uncontrolled blood glucose swings in themselves—Will I go high from having to eat more? Will I go low from "sharing" with my baby? You may be relieved to find out that women with diabetes can and do breastfeed successfully, and your milk may even reduce the chances of passing diabetes on to your baby.

Breast Benefits

Clinical studies suggest that women who have gestational diabetes in pregnancy and go on to breastfeed their child for at least three months experience improved glucose tolerance and pancreatic beta cell function, which may lessen their chances of developing type 2 diabetes later in life. Breastfeeding may also be protective for the children of at-risk type

2 populations. Several studies have also found that Native American mothers who breastfeed reduce the risk of their children developing the disease.

Safety Measures

Taking insulin does not threaten the health of your breastfeeding infant. However, women who take medication to control their type 2 diabetes need to consult with their doctor, as some drugs pass into breastmilk. Your doctor can help you weigh the benefits of breastfeeding against any risks medication might pose. In some cases, he may be able to prescribe an alternative drug. If you are pregnant and plan on breastfeeding your child, you should discuss these issues with your doctor now, so you are both prepared once the baby arrives.

Breastfeeding can be hard work (especially for first-time moms), and when you're trying to balance it with the demanding occupation of new motherhood, the associated stress and fatigue can do a number on your control. The hormonal changes associated with breastfeeding and the postpartum period can also cause highs and lows (although in some women, this shift may improve sugar levels). As you may have guessed already, checking your glucose levels often and working with your doctor are the best ways to stay on track during this hectic time.

Avoiding Hypos

You'll need extra calories and fluid in your daily diet to keep your milk supply and your energy level up. If you haven't seen your dietitian lately, now is the time to go in for a refresher appointment. She can help you to create a meal plan that can promote successful breastfeeding, reasonable postpartum weight loss, and good diabetes control.

Not surprisingly, nursing can cause a drop in blood sugar levels in women who take insulin and certain oral medications. To avoid going low, have a protein/carb snack and something to drink either before or during nursing. This is particularly important for those middle-of-the-night feedings. Keep some quick and easy snacks on hand where you nurse, or consider setting up a minifridge with a childproof lock. Glucose tablets or other fast-acting sugars should be easily accessible in case of a low, and a meter should be stowed within reach to make checking levels easy (but don't forget to store it more securely once the baby is old enough to get around, which will be sooner than you think).

FACT

As with mothers without diabetes, there is no set timetable for weaning. However, when you and baby decide it is time, it should be done gradually, if possible. In addition to stirring up the hormones again, you may have to adjust your diet to stay consistent with your control. Talk to your dietitian about your particular needs.

When It's Time for Menopause

The big change in your early fifties usually brings about changes in your diabetes treatment needs as well. In addition to the mood swings, the slowdown of estrogen and progesterone production can put your blood sugars on a swing of their own. In fact, you may actually start experiencing these symptoms well before menopause, in the proceeding period known as perimenopause that starts anywhere from ages forty-five to fifty-five (average age being forty-seven).

How Menopause Affects Diabetes

Lower estrogen levels may increase insulin resistance in type 2 women, while lower progesterone levels have the opposite effect, increasing insulin sensitivity. For this reason, one woman's glycemic (or blood sugar) response to menopause can be very different from another's. The best way to figure out what's going on with you is to test your glucose levels frequently and work closely with your doctor.

The ADA reports that, on average, most women require less medication for type 2 diabetes after menopause. However, weight gain, which occurs in response to a slowing metabolism and declining estrogen levels, may offset this benefit. So can inactivity (another reason to keep on track with fitness at any and every age).

According to the Mayo Clinic, women with diabetes who are postmenopausal have a risk of heart attack or stroke that is three times that of their peers without diabetes. One solution for some women be hormone replacement therapy (HRT), available in a pill, patch, cream, or vaginal insert.

HRT: Risks Versus Benefits

Whether or not to take hormone replacement therapy (HRT) to combat some of the menopausal problems unique to women with diabetes is very much an individual decision, based on your own medical situation and cardiovascular risk profile. Oral estrogen therapy may improve your cholesterol profile by lowering your LDL (bad) and raising your HDL (good) cholesterol, but it has also been found to increase triglyceride levels, which ups cardiovascular risk.

Some studies have found that low-dose, continuous transdermal HRT may improve fasting glucose levels and decrease total cholesterol in postmenopausal women with type 2 diabetes. However, these trials were small and further large-scale, long-term study of this therapy is needed. It's important that you discuss the full risks and benefits of HRT with your doctor before making a treatment decision.

Female Sexual Dysfunction

In this post-Viagra age, the American public is well aware of the problems of male impotence. But female sexual dysfunction and arousal problems remain a less publicized cause. You may be surprised to learn that according to results of a national study published in the *Journal of the American Medical Association*, sexual dysfunction was actually more prevalent in women than in men (43 versus 31 percent).

Uncontrolled blood sugar levels affect arousal, performance, and overall well-being. High blood sugars trigger yeast infections and vaginal irritation. In addition, vascular damage can restrict blood flow to the vagina, causing lubrication problems. Women who have neuropathy that affects the genital area, the reproductive organs, and/or the vagina may have difficulty achieving arousal and orgasm.

Psychological Factors

Sometimes the problem is more psychological than physical. The less-romantic aspects of treatment, such as needing to do a blood sugar check before sex, can make some women self-conscious and less likely to initiate or participate in it.

Fear may be a factor in your ability to let go and relax, as well. You may be afraid that the physical exertion of sex will trigger hypoglycemia. Taking the same precautions you do for exercise will usually prevent blood sugar lows. However, make sure your partner knows that in the unlikely event that you do lose consciousness, it wasn't his performance that did it. Give him a briefing on when to seek emergency medical care for you.

Other Culprits

A number of other issues can contribute to sexual difficulties in women with diabetes:

- Certain medications (e.g., antidepressants, hypertension medications)
- Menopause (low estrogen levels can cause vaginal dryness)
- Vaginismus (a tightening of the vaginal walls that may make sex painful)
- Excess weight or obesity—overweight women may feel self-conscious and unattractive

Treatments

Therapy and/or medication may help you overcome depression. Make sure you talk to your doctor about the possible sexual side effects of any antidepressant she may prescribe. Some drugs, such as Wellbutrin (bupro-prion), have lower risks of sexual side effects and may be preferred.

If low estrogen levels are at the root of vaginal dryness problems, hormone replacement therapy can sometimes alleviate this problem, but it should be prescribed with caution in some women. Over-the-counter lubricants are also available to ease dryness and painful penetration. If your partner uses condoms, stick with water-based lubricants, as oil-based products react with latex and can encourage breakage. Medical devices designed to stimulate blood flow in the genitals and increase lubrication may also be prescribed. Your gynecologist or urologist can tell you more about these options.

As with most complications related to diabetes, adjustments to your diet, medication, and exercise routines may improve both your diabetes and your sex drive.

ALERT

If you're suffering from sexual dysfunction, you need to talk to your doctor about the problem. In some cases, it may be a sign of a diabetic complication that needs treatment. Even if it is something more benign, you owe it to yourself to find a solution. Don't let the embarrassment stop you—your doctor is there to help.

How Women Cope

Managing chronic illness day in and day out can be stressful and emotionally draining. If you're newly diagnosed, you're trying to get your mental and physical bearings to figure out your own path to diabetes control. You've been thrown into this disease headfirst, and, even with the best diabetes care team guiding you, these early days can be stressful, scary, and anxious. In a worst-case scenario, you may have been handed a diagnosis, a one-size-fits-all "diabetic diet" and/or prescription, and shown the door to figure things out on your own.

Dealing with Depression

People with diabetes are twice as likely to suffer from depression than the general population, and women with diabetes are more likely to experience depression than men are. It's normal to experience some depressive symptoms at diagnosis, but when depression starts to interfere with everyday life and you start to lose interest in things you used to enjoy, you may be experiencing a major depressive episode.

Depression distracts you from proper diabetes care, and clinical studies have shown that people with diabetes who are depressed have higher blood sugar levels and a higher incidence of microvascular and macrovascular diabetic complications. Add poor control, and the symptoms and psychological impact of knowing you aren't doing well with your diabetes care can make you even more depressed, resulting in a downward spiral of diabetes highs and emotional lows.

Diabetes can be a heavy load to carry, and depression seems to double that weight. Ignore either and they'll only get worse. You don't have to suffer in silence. Let your doctor know if you're experiencing signs of depression. Therapy or antidepressant medication may be options for you.

ESSENTIAL

Wearing an insulin pump can present unique challenges in the bedroom. If you decide you want to disconnect it before sex, be sure to take into account the amount of time you are off the pump and the exertion factor, and adjust accordingly once you're pumping again. Others prefer to stay hooked up and use a longer infusion or tubing set.

Weighty Issues

For women with type 2 diabetes, who often have weight problems, negative body image is a prevalent problem. Sometimes, the start of insulin therapy can compound the problem, resulting in unwanted weight gain. This can be a source of major frustration and may also take a take a toll on self-esteem, particularly in the teen years.

FACT

A *Journal of the American Medical Association* study reported that women who watch twenty hours or more of television each week are more likely to experience obesity, diabetes, and other health risks. Researchers found that every two hours spent watching television was associated with a 14 percent increase in diabetes risk. Several other studies have confirmed these findings.

Aside from contributing to depression, a poor self-image can hinder your sex life and be a source of stress and anxiety. Living a fit and active lifestyle should not be identified with being supermodel skinny. Accepting yourself—at any size—is important to your physical and psychological well-being.

Sometimes weight problems can feel so insurmountable that women are hesitant to take that first step forward for fear of failure. Soon they find themselves in an endless cycle of bingeing, bad feelings, and sky-high blood sugar levels. Consequently, self-esteem plummets along with diabetes control. Yes, weight loss can be hard, but you don't have to go it alone. Your doctor, registered dietitian, and diabetes care team are all there to help you succeed.

CHAPTER 16

Men and Diabetes

Men with diabetes face unique challenges of their own. Men may be less apt to express any feelings of anxiety or depression they're facing while trying to come to terms with the disease, and one of the most prevalent complications in men with diabetes—erectile dysfunction—is definitely an emotionally loaded issue. But while men face a higher risk of certain diabetic complications, they are more likely to report feeling in control of their diabetes and on top of their treatment, both big benefits in dealing with chronic disease.

At Puberty

The hormonal changes that accompany puberty actually increase insulin resistance in both boys and girls. In boys, adiponectin, a hormone that regulates glucose and insulin, takes a marked drop in puberty. And boys who are overweight or obese have the added problem of lower testosterone levels, which also contributes to insulin resistance.

Puberty typically starts around age ten for most boys, but weight problems sometimes delay the onset of puberty (unlike in overweight girls, for which puberty may hit much earlier).

A Turbulent Time

Puberty is a time of separation from parents and a growing emphasis on social relationships—creating a separate social identity is paramount. Boys who may have depended on their parents for guidance on diabetes care may start taking more responsibility for their own care. Likewise, parents must learn to hand over the reins of diabetes control, at least partially, to allow their child to mature emotionally as well as physically.

FACT

The amount of time teenage boys spend in front of a computer, video game, or TV screen can impact their health. Studies have associated prolonged (two-plus hours a day) screen time with abnormal insulin levels and insulin resistance in adolescent boys.

However, the social pressures of puberty can also push young men in the opposite direction of ignoring their diabetes for the sake of being more like their peers. Drug and alcohol use—experimental or otherwise—can also become a problem during this time of life. American adolescent males are statistically more likely to drink alcohol and take illicit drugs than are girls of a similar age. In a national 2011 CDC survey of high school students, nearly 24 percent of boys between the ages of twelve and twenty report recent binge drinking (defined as five or more drinks of alcohol in a single sitting in the past month).

Because alcohol can impair treatment judgment and trigger a potentially dangerous hypoglycemic episode, it's important that boys (and girls) with diabetes are educated about the special risks they face with alcohol and drug use. Even though "Just Say No" is good advice, realistically, many youths may not follow it. Especially during adolescence, kids need to know what precautions are necessary if they do drink.

FACT

There are 13 million adult males with diabetes in the United States—that's 11.8 percent of all American men. An estimated one-third of these men are not even aware that they have diabetes.

Changes in Testosterone Levels

Testosterone levels in men begin to decrease starting around age forty, eventually leading to what some have called "male menopause" or andropause, which brings with it an increased cardiovascular risk, loss of muscle and bone mass, and a waning libido. Other signs of declining testosterone can include lower sperm count, body hair loss, and even hot flashes.

Men with diabetes tend to have a lower-than-average testosterone level. The classic "apple-shaped" body of type 2 diabetes, also known variously as intra-abdominal fat or central fat storage (or, in more familiar terms, beer belly), is associated with low testosterone levels in men. Also known as hypogonadism, this condition is also associated with high levels of circulating insulin (hyperinsulinemia) and increased insulin resistance. Low levels of the hormone are thought to affect glucose metabolism; some studies have linked improved glucose tolerance with testosterone replacement therapy.

HRT—Not Just for Women

Testosterone replacement therapy, in the form of injections or a transdermal (through the skin) gel or patch, may be beneficial to many older men with low testosterone levels. The jury is still out on whether this therapy can slow or even prevent the onset of type 2 diabetes by inhibiting intra-abdominal fat accumulation.

Sexuality and Impotence

Impotence—the failure to get or maintain an erection—is one of the most common and most distressing side effects of diabetes. Between 20 and 71 percent of men with diabetes have experienced impotence at some point since diagnosis. If you've had problems with erectile dysfunction (ED), you are not alone.

Some men delay getting treatment for ED because of embarrassment or self-consciousness, but ED can be the first sign of a more serious underlying diabetes complication, such as cardiovascular disease or neuropathy, so it's important not to ignore it or delay medical attention for the problem. Your doctor is quite used to dealing with impotence issues and has a variety of treatment options at his disposal.

FACT

Smoking can contribute to erectile dysfunction by causing constriction of blood vessels, leading to hypertension. Nicotine also promotes the growth of artery-clogging cholesterol plaques, which contribute to high blood pressure.

What Causes ED

There are many possible causes of male impotence, ranging from surgery to smoking; the following are most likely to affect men with diabetes:

- **Medications.** Drugs such as high blood pressure medications, certain antidepressants, and tranquilizers can trigger episodes of impotence. Your doctor may be able to adjust your dosage or substitute another medication.
- **Neuropathy.** Nerve damage to the penis itself or to the autonomic nervous system may be the cause of ED.
- **Cardiovascular disease.** Clogged arteries, especially those that feed the corpora cavernosa (the spongy vascular tissue of the penis) can impair circulation enough to inhibit an erection.
- **Psychological issues.** Depression, anxiety, and stress related to diabetes management can inhibit sexual performance.

Treatment Options

There are a number of options available for treating ED, including medication, vacuum devices, surgery, and psychosocial therapy. The least-invasive nonpharmaceutical method of treatment is a mechanical vacuum device. A cylinder is placed over the length of the penis and a hand-operated vacuum pump is used to remove the air from the cylinder, creating a vacuum and pulling blood into the penis to create an erection. Once erection has been achieved, it is sustained with the use of a tension ring placed at the base of the penis.

ALERT

Men who use nitroglycerin ointment (applied to the penis) to treat ED should wear a condom during intercourse. Nitroglycerin is absorbed through the skin, including the vagina, and can cause a headache or other symptoms in your partner. Of course, wearing a condom is always recommended if you aren't involved in a long-term, monogamous relationship.

The thought of a hypodermic syringe anywhere near your groin area might send shivers down your spine, but some men with ED caused by neuropathy can be helped with one of several drugs that are injected directly into the penis (papaverine hydrochloride, phentolamine, and alprostadil, also known as Caverject or Edex) to dilate, or widen, blood vessels and cause an erection. Alprostadil is also available in a suppository (Medicated Urethral System for Injection, or MUSE) that can be inserted into the urethra, a more palatable choice for some men. Topical vasodilators (e.g., nitroglycerin ointment, minoxidil)—medications that are rubbed on the penis to improve blood flow—may also be an option, but reports of their success are mixed.

Several oral medications have been approved for the treatment of erectile dysfunction, including sildenafil citrate (Viagra), vardenafil (Levitra; Staxyn), and tadalafil (Cialis). These drugs have helped millions of men with erectile dysfunction problems since Viagra—the first—was released in 1998. And the latest, avanafil (Stendra), was approved by the FDA in early 2012.

These drugs are taken before sexual activity and work by enhancing the effects of nitric oxide on the body, which dilates blood vessels and acts as a smooth-muscle relaxant. This improves blood flow to the penis and facilitates an erection when sexual arousal occurs. One potential drawback of Viagra and Levitra is the need to take these drugs about an hour before sex; if you're a spur-of-the-moment kind of guy, you'll need a new strategy. Cialis, on the other hand, works for up to thirty-six hours, giving you a larger window of opportunity. And Stendra, the newest of the ED drugs, starts working in as little as fifteen to thirty minutes.

QUESTION

I have a heart condition. Can sex make it worse?
Unless your heart is severely impaired (i.e., congestive heart failure), there is really very little risk of normal sexual activity triggering a heart attack. Halting all exercise—and sex—is probably one of the worst things for hypertension. A chat with your doctor about your concerns will help you ease your mind about sex.

Insertion of a penile implant, or treatment and repair of arterial and venous damage related to ED, are more invasive options to treat impotence. Your doctor can discuss treatment options that are right for you.

If your impotence is rooted in depression, anxiety, or other emotional issues, your doctor may refer you to a counselor, psychiatrist, or psychologist for help in sorting through it all. A couple's therapist may also be helpful for uncovering sources of marital tension.

Diabetes and Fertility

Men with long-term, uncontrolled diabetes can suffer nerve damage that causes a condition known as retrograde ejaculation—where semen is deposited into the urinary bladder instead of being ejaculated out the head of the penis. This happens because the small muscle that controls the passageway into the bladder becomes damaged and doesn't close as it should during climax, so sperm is rerouted into the bladder.

Some men may have reduced ejaculate as a result of this condition, while others may not ejaculate at all. The latter is referred to as dry climax. Retrograde ejaculation can be a cause of male infertility, and if it is caused by neuropathy it cannot be surgically corrected at this point in time. If you have symptoms of the condition, you should talk to your doctor about a referral to a urologist. Couples who have trouble conceiving due to retrograde ejaculation should see a fertility specialist. Assisted reproduction may be a possibility by retrieving sperm through a bladder-washing procedure and using it to inseminate your partner artificially.

Complications: Gender Bias?

While diabetes crosses all age, racial, and gender lines, it does seem to show some questionably preferential treatment to men in the distribution of certain diabetic complications. For example, the ADA reports that men diagnosed with diabetes before age thirty tend to develop retinopathy more rapidly than their female counterparts. And among people with diabetes, first heart attacks are more likely to be fatal in men than women.

Men with type 2 diabetes are more likely to develop coronary artery disease (CAD) than their male counterparts without diabetes. They are also more likely to have additional CAD risk factors, such as high triglycerides, high blood pressure, and obesity.

How Men Cope

A ten-year study of gender differences in attitudes toward diabetes at the Johns Hopkins Diabetes Center found that men tended to have more positive attitudes toward and greater acceptance of their diabetes than do women with the disease. Accordingly, they also tended to rate their quality of life higher. The study also found that men were more accepting of their treatment regimen, and were less likely to miss work or leisure activities due to their diabetes.

FACT

According to the ADA, amputation rates are 1.4 to 2.7 times higher in men than in women. However, with proper preventive foot care and wound treatment, the risk drops dramatically.

Perhaps reflecting traditional "woman as caretaker" gender roles, men with diabetes were also satisfied with the level of emotional support they received from their wives or partners, who were more likely to accompany them to appointments and diabetes education classes than were male partners or husbands of women with diabetes. Interestingly, while men with diabetes did not miss work or leisure activities, their wives were more likely to have to take time off attributed to their husband's disease, yet these women reported feeling less anxious about the long-term impact of the disease on their family than did the husbands of women with diabetes.

Men in this study also reported more control over their diabetes in terms of lower A1C levels, better self-reported nutritional care and insulin adherence, and fewer complications than women.

ESSENTIAL

When things aren't going well with diabetes management, some men can take it as a sign of personal failure, and the resulting stress can make the situation worse. Think of erratic blood glucose levels as a challenge rather than a fault. Use your health care team and your support system to figure out the mystery.

Men and Stress Management

But what about when things don't go right? Problems with erratic blood sugar levels and elusive control can cause stress levels to climb. This leads to a vicious circle of control issues, as high stress produces high blood sugar levels, high blood pressure, and further anxiety about your ability to manage your disease.

Studies have proved that stress management training can improve long-term blood sugar control, thus reducing your risk of complications. They have also demonstrated that daily practice of stress management techniques by men with heart disease can slash their risk of cardiovascular incidents like surgery and heart attack in comparison with those who used exercise or standard therapy (medication and monitoring).

CHAPTER 17

Aging Well with Diabetes

Twenty-seven percent of Americans age sixty-five and older, or nearly eleven million seniors, are living with diabetes. And a staggering half of all people in this age group have prediabetes. Additional health challenges, including those that limit mobility and affect memory, can make diabetes increasingly hard to manage as you age. You may also face a variety of financial, social, and family changes, and all can have a profound impact on your diabetes care. Fortunately, there are many treatment strategies and programs available to make things easier.

Senior Lifestyle Challenges

As you age, diabetes management can get more challenging on several fronts. Health and family circumstances may make you more reliant on others. A retirement or other career transition may mean that you are living on a stricter fixed budget. And your social support system may be limited as family and friends also age and make their own transitions.

Yet managing your diabetes is even more important as you reach this phase in your life. Age brings about additional health issues that can complicate diabetes care. And this often means a myriad of treatments, doctor's appointments, and prescription drugs to deal with.

Fortunately, there is financial, transportation, and social assistance available for many seniors. And by using these resources, you can stay healthy, happy, and in control of your diabetes.

Finances

If you are living on a fixed income due to retirement or disability, the cost of diabetes care can become a burden. Skimping on medication, needed doctor's visits, and healthy food choices to make ends meet can have an impact on your blood sugar control and overall health.

Medicare can help pay for diabetes supplies, exams, and equipment like shoes and blood sugar meters. You can call 1-800-Medicare to find out what you qualify for. Medicare benefits are also covered in greater detail later in this chapter.

Mobility

Arthritis and other age-related conditions can affect your ability to get the exercise you need. According to the CDC, by the age of seventy-five, one in three men and half of all women are inactive. And this lack of physical activity has a direct effect on diabetes control and heart health.

In addition, age-related health problems such as worsening vision and poor dexterity can impact your ability to drive. This limited access to transportation can make it hard to get to doctor's appointments and to have timely access to pick up prescriptions and purchase fresh food.

If you no longer drive and your community does not have public transportation, there are often options for you. Call your town hall, senior center, or local church to ask about senior citizen transit programs they may sponsor. In addition, these organizations may know of meal delivery services (e.g., "Meals on Wheels") that you could be eligible for.

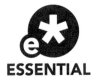

ESSENTIAL

The United States Department of Agriculture provides low-income seniors with access to healthy foods through the Supplemental Nutrition Assistance Program (SNAP). You can get information on SNAP by calling 1-800-221-5689. You can also search for food banks in your area at *feedingamerica.org*.

Isolation and Social Support

Seniors who lack social or family support may feel isolated. Diabetes already raises the risk of depression, and that risk is magnified in older adults who feel "cut off" from the world. One University of Florida study found that seniors with type 2 diabetes were twice as likely to suffer from depression as those their age without diabetes. Depression can in turn lead to a decline in good diabetes care.

If your family and friends are far away, stay in touch regularly via phone or computers. And try to build a new local support system by getting active in your community. Volunteering at a local school, church, or hospital is one way to start. A local senior center can also be a great place to connect with others.

If you are experiencing signs of depression, such as difficulty sleeping, changes in appetite, profound sadness, and a loss of pleasure in activities you used to enjoy, talk to your doctor. Depression can be easily treated and your diabetes control and overall quality of life will improve with that treatment.

Staying Sharp: Cognition and Memory

Everyone has the occasional "where'd I put the car keys?" moment. These blips in our memory are normal and typically aren't a sign of any deeper problems. But when these start to lapse into more serious forgetfulness, like leaving the stove on or forgetting people or places, they should be evaluated by a doctor.

People with type 2 have an increased risk for developing mild cognitive impairment, dementia, and Alzheimer's disease. The damage that chronic uncontrolled blood sugar can do to the small blood vessels that feed the brain can cause something known as vascular dementia.

And in recent years, researchers have found a link between high blood sugars and the brain plaques that develop in Alzheimer's; it is possible that there may be a genetic link between diabetes and Alzheimer's.

If you're experiencing memory or cognition problems, particularly if you are taking insulin, your doctor may choose to target a slightly higher A1C goal for you. This is in part because frequent episodes of hypoglycemia, or low blood sugar, have been associated with cognitive problems in seniors with type 2.

Aside from doing your best to meet the blood sugar targets your doctor has set for you, you can also take other steps to stay sharp. Brain-bending puzzles and word games like Sudoku, Scrabble, and crosswords can help keep your mental muscle toned. Use alarms, planners, and visual reminders to stay on top of daily tasks you may tend to forget, such as taking your medicines.

Getting Past Medication Barriers

More than 76 percent of Americans over age sixty use two or more prescription drugs, and 37 percent use five or more. More prescriptions means more pills to remember to take, medication instructions to understand, and side effects and interactions to manage. Add over-the-counter medicines and supplements to the mix and the task becomes even bigger. There's a word for this challenge—polypharmacy.

ALERT

Multiple prescriptions from different doctors can lead to drug interactions and prescribing errors without careful attention. When you get a new prescription, make sure your doctor knows the other medicines you are taking. Getting all your prescriptions filled at a single drugstore that routinely checks for these types of interactions may also help prevent problems.

In addition to managing all of these medications, there's the matter of paying for them, keeping on schedule, and working through side effects.

Remembering, and Understanding, It All

If you are taking more than one or two prescription drugs, it can be difficult to keep track of them all. Which one gets taken with food, and which one on an empty stomach? Which pills should never be taken together? And can you safely add over-the-counter pain relievers or cold medicine to the mix?

When you get a new prescription, ask your doctor about the dose and when and how it should be taken. If you see more than one physician that prescribes drugs for you, it's very important that they are aware of ALL the medicines you are taking. It's a good idea to bring all of your prescription medicines, along with any over-the-counter drugs or supplements you take regularly, to your doctor's appointments. Include the original packaging and labels.

Reviewing your medicines with your doctor or diabetes educator at least once a year is a good practice to ensure you're taking everything correctly and to avoid any drug interactions.

Of course, understanding how to take your drugs is only half the battle. The bigger challenge may be remembering to take them on time, and the more you have, the tougher it can be. Using a pill organizer is a great first step. These run the gamut from simple plastic boxes to sophisticated electronic dispensers, and are available at your local pharmacy. Audible alarms, from cell or smartphone reminders to a simple kitchen timer, can also help jog your memory.

Many people find that a written medication diary is a helpful tool to keep track of their daily drug routine. This can be as simple as handwritten notes in a calendar or daily organizer. Or a list of drugs in a notebook to check off daily. Experiment with different memory aids and see what works well for you.

The High Cost of Health

Prescription drugs can be expensive, and the more you have, the bigger the financial burden. When starting a new drug, ask your doctor for some samples to get you started. There may also be a cheaper generic option for the drug, so ask your doctor or pharmacist about this as well.

If the cost isn't covered by your health insurance or Medicare and remains out of your reach, the drug manufacturer may be able to help. Many pharmaceutical companies have patient assistance programs that provide needed drugs at little to no cost. Call the Partnership for Prescription Assistance at 1-888-4PPA-NOW (1-888-477-2669) to get more information.

Sticking Out Side Effects

Often, drugs come with side effects that can make sticking it out rough. For example, the widely prescribed type 2 diabetes drug metformin is well known for its gastrointestinal side effects. It can take weeks to months for a drug to reach its full therapeutic potential, so make sure you've given it a fair chance.

Instead of stopping outright, call your doctor. A dose adjustment can often help. By titrating the drug, or starting with a small amount that is gradually increased over time, side effects can be minimized. And typically they will lessen and often disappear over time.

Mobility and Exercise

Your need to keep moving does not decline with age. In fact, regular exercise can actually help keep seniors flexible and mobile, and helps improves balance (which may prevent falls). It can also counteract the natural decline in muscle strength that occurs with age. And of course, aerobic and resistance exercise combined continues to be key in improving blood sugar control.

For many seniors, walking is an easy, low cost, low impact way to stay fit. Daily walks with family, friends, or pets can keep you motivated. Many gyms, community centers, and health care plans also offer "seniors only" workout programs. The nationally recognized program Silver Sneakers offers classes through Medicare health plans in many areas. Call 1-888-423-4632 to find out about options in your area.

For those with disabilities, or with joint pain and arthritis that make high impact exercise difficult, there are low impact ways to work a heart-pumping aerobic workout into your day. Swimming and water workouts can be good aerobic and resistance exercise choices. Chair exercise programs are also an excellent choice for the disabled. Before starting any fitness program, get medical clearance from your doctor.

Medicare and You

If you are age sixty-five or older, you are probably familiar with Medicare. This government subsidized health insurance program makes care affordable for millions of seniors. It also provides quite a few diabetes benefits that you may not be aware of.

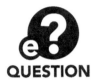

QUESTION

My husband has diabetic kidney disease and will be starting on dialysis. His doctor said he's eligible for Medicare but he's only sixty-three. Is that right?
The doctor is right. In some cases, Medicare coverage kicks in before age sixty-five. Certain disabilities and health conditions provide earlier coverage. End-stage renal disease (ESRD), or kidney failure, is one of these.

Your particular coverage will depend on which Medicare programs you have enrolled in, but the following is a brief overview of diabetes benefits that are available in two common enrollment plans—Part B and Part D.

If you have a Medicare Advantage (or Part C) program, which is a Medicare program administered through a private insurer, you may have different diabetes benefits and requirements for coverage. Check with your plan administrator to make sure you are making the most of your Medicare coverage.

Part B Diabetes Coverage

Medicare Part B is the health insurance component of Medicare that covers doctor's visits, outpatient care, and durable medical equipment. It does not cover hospital stays, which are included in Medicare Part A. Many of your diabetes benefits, including testing equipment and supplies and diabetes education, are covered by Part B.

You must enroll in Part B in the seven-month window surrounding your sixty-fifth birthday (starting three months before and closing three months after your birthday month). If you fail to sign up at this time, Medicare will charge you a late enrollment penalty.

Following is a list of diabetes benefits covered by Medicare Part B. Unless otherwise noted, you are responsible for 20 percent of the cost (Medicare pays the remaining 80 percent). You must meet your Part B deductible first for all of these benefits except the welcome exam and the immunizations.

- **"Welcome to Medicare" exam.** This comprehensive physical examination includes a review of your entire health history and referrals for other screenings, if necessary. But it must take place within a year of your enrollment to Medicare. If you are still within your eligibility period and haven't taken advantage of this benefit, call to schedule yours now.
- **Diabetes education and medical nutrition therapy.** Medicare covers diabetes self-management training from a certified diabetes educator or other approved program as long as you have a written order from your doctor. The same goes for a visit with a registered dietitian to create a dietary plan.
- **Blood sugar testing supplies.** A blood sugar monitor, lancing device, lancets, and test strips are covered by Medicare. The number of test strips Part B will cover may be limited. In general, patients on insulin get the most coverage, of up to 100 test strips a month. But your doctor can approve more strips and lancets as "medically necessary."
- **Glaucoma and foot screenings.** If you have peripheral neuropathy, Medicare will cover a foot exam every six months. Glaucoma screenings are covered annually.
- **Therapeutic shoes or inserts.** If you have diabetes-related foot problems and your podiatrist prescribes custom therapeutic shoes or inserts, Medicare will cover them as long as they are fitted by a qualified professional (e.g., orthotist, prosthetist, pedorthist).
- **Influenza and pneumococcal vaccines.** Annual vaccinations are covered, free of charge (no deductible or co-pay).

FACT

While Medicare Part B does provide coverage for insulin pumps, patients must meet fairly strict clinical guidelines to be eligible. These include undergoing blood tests for c-peptide levels, a history of multiple daily injections, and completing diabetes self-management classes. Medicare also requires a documented medical need, such as an A1C over 7 percent.

Remember that in order to receive coverage for these items, you'll need a prescription from your doctor, even for items that don't require a prescription to purchase, such as test strips and lancets. Prescriptions for test strips should include your doctor's directions for how many times you test per day, and whether or not you use insulin.

Part D Prescription Drugs

Medicare Part D covers oral and injectable diabetes drugs, including insulin. If you use an insulin pump that is *not* covered by Medicare, however, the insulin you use to fill it will not be covered.

Any supplies you require to inject insulin, such as syringes, pens, and alcohol swabs, are also covered by Medicare Part D. A Part D deductible may apply for all these drugs and insulin supplies; if you are unsure of your Part D benefits, talk to your plan administrator or call 1-800-MEDICARE (1-800-633-4227).

Caring for a Parent with Diabetes

If your elderly mom or dad is living independently and diabetes has become a health issue for them, it's natural to be concerned and want to help. And there are many ways to do so while still giving them autonomy over their own health.

Empowering your parent is important because diabetes is a disease that requires good self-management. No caregiver, no matter how hard they try, can control blood sugar for the person living with diabetes. Diabetes is more than just taking your medicine on time, even for older adults. You also need good exercise, eating, stress management, and sleep habits to stay on top of it—all behaviors that must be managed by the patient.

Communicate, Don't Dictate

Parent/child role reversal is hard to resist when an older parent develops a chronic health condition. The best way to avoid this situation is to keep the lines of communication open. Ask your parent how you can help her stay healthy. This may run the gamut from driving to and attending doctor's appointments with her to just being an occasional sounding board for her concerns. It's okay to make suggestions, but accept the answers she gives you and don't assume responsibilities she may not want to share.

ALERT

If your older parent lives alone, make sure he is prepared for an emergency. Put a list of emergency phone numbers next to every phone, and program the most important ones into his cell phone if he has one. Encourage the use of medical identification, and look into the possibility of an emergency medical response service, so the push of a button will bring him assistance.

Remember that your parent is an adult with the right to make her own decisions. Your job is to support her. This means making sure she fully understands the options in front of her for treatment. When she is put on a new medicine or treatment routine, periodically ask her how it's going, and encourage a phone call to the doctor's office if things aren't progressing as expected. You may also suggest helping your parent keep a list of questions she has about her diabetes care that she can bring to her next appointment.

Avoiding Caregiver Burnout

It may be tempting to try and do it all for your mom or dad, especially if you live nearby, but this isn't good for either of you. It doesn't allow your parent full ownership over his diabetes and his own care, and it can become extremely stressful for you.

In some cases, taking on a larger share of your parent's diabetes responsibilities is unavoidable. If your parent still lives independently, but no longer drives and has limited mobility, you may be juggling quite a few care and home tasks. If financially possible, home visits from a health care nurse are an excellent way to reduce stress and also give your parent a new and compassionate face to spend some time with.

You should also enlist the help of family, neighbors, and friends and set a regular visitation schedule for your mom or dad. It's just as important for your parent not to feel isolated and shut in as it is for you to know he or she has a larger community to rely on.

CHAPTER 18

Diabetes, Emotions, and Relationships

In addition to blood sugar highs and lows, diabetes triggers emotional ups and downs that can be just as unpredictable and severe. And because the disease is life altering, it has a significant emotional impact on not just the patient, but on everyone who lives with and cares for her or him. Learning healthy coping techniques will help you and those around you live a healthier, happier life.

Dealing with Diagnosis

Dealing with a diabetes diagnosis has been compared to coping with the grief of death. Diagnosis marks the loss of life as you knew it. It's normal to grieve your old "healthy" life, even if you weren't feeling well before getting the diabetes label. Denial, anger, bargaining, depression, and acceptance are all part of the process.

The Dangers of Denial

The first of these can be the hardest and most damaging in diabetes. Many people choose simply to ignore that they have the disease, continuing on as if it didn't exist. The problem with this (non)coping approach is the long-term consequences of uncontrolled blood glucose. By the time they do come to terms with denial and are ready to treat their diabetes, serious complications may be on their way.

Some newly diagnosed patients will acknowledge their feelings of denial. Recognition is a good sign that in the back of your mind you know you must move forward. As long as you're willing to follow your doctor's orders for the time being, even if you haven't fully accepted the disease, denial is a normal part of the process.

ALERT

For patients who reject both the diagnosis and the treatment, the situation can become a dangerous one. Sometimes it takes a blood sugar emergency that lands them in the hospital or the development of diabetic complications for them to realize that they do, indeed, have diabetes.

Reaching acceptance can be a difficult, rocky road. Many people need the help of a therapist or counselor to get there. A health psychologist who has specialized training in the intricate psychological, biological, and social relationships between physical illness and mental health can be helpful in sorting through coping issues.

Personality Types and Diabetes Success

Studies have shown that your personality type may influence the kind of "diabetes manager" you are. Research out of the University of Washington found that people with an "independent" personality type, associated with self-reliance, are actually worse managers of their diabetes than those with an "interactive" personality type. The reason? Those with an interactive personality type were more collaborative, and therefore more likely to ask for help when they needed it. And because the health care system in general is a collaborative one, and diabetes care specifically involves collaboration among the patient and an extended network of care providers, interactive personalities are more successful there.

Independent personalities had a 33 percent increased risk of dying over the five-year study period. Hallmark characteristics of this personality type are a need to "do it all" themselves, a general mistrust of others, and a reluctance to ask others for assistance when they needed it.

That doesn't mean you need give up all hope if you consider yourself the independent type. Self-awareness that you may not be able to "do it all" when it comes to diabetes is the first step. And finding a diabetes doctor you really trust is particularly important.

The Emotional Roller Coaster

Although acceptance is an important step in getting on track to diabetes control, it isn't a guarantee of ongoing inner peace. Periods of difficult control and high blood sugars can also bring devastating emotional lows, which can in turn make blood sugar levels rise even farther and start a self-perpetuating cycle of physical and psychological deterioration. Learn to recognize the signs of emotional pitfalls like depression, anger, guilt, and stress so you can take the appropriate steps to stop this downward spiral before it starts.

Depression

Up to 30 percent of people with diabetes also suffer from symptoms of depression, and people with diabetes are twice as likely to become clinically depressed than are those without diabetes. Occasional sadness, fear, and uncertainty are normal in diabetes, but when they start affecting your everyday enjoyment of life and interfering with proper self-care, they may be something more than just a passing emotional downturn.

FACT

Signs of a depressive disorder include weight loss, insomnia (too little sleep) or hypersomnia (too much sleep), irritability or agitation, fatigue, feelings of guilt or worthlessness, inability to concentrate, and recurrent thoughts of death or suicide.

Depression can be treated with therapy and/or antidepressant medication, so there's no reason to suffer needlessly. Here are a few other points that may help you deal with depression:

- **Knowledge is power.** Fear of the unknown can feed your depression. If you haven't already done so, start educating yourself about your disease.
- **Seek support.** Draw on the experience and emotional comfort of your family, friends, spiritual community, health care team, and others with diabetes.
- **Keep perfection in perspective.** Reward your successes, big or small, and try to see your stumbles as learning experiences rather than failures.
- **Keep moving.** Try to push yourself to take a brisk walk daily. Exercise raises your level of endorphins, a natural mood booster.

Anger Management

You have diabetes and you're foot-stamping, wall-slamming, screaming, steaming mad about it. Now the question is, what do you do with all that pent-up hostility? Do you focus it on beating the snot out of that damned disease through aggressive diabetes control, or do you turn it outward at the world and push away your family and care providers in the process?

Anger is an understandable reaction to diabetes, and it can be a good motivational tool if used appropriately. However, if it's becoming a barrier to your care and your relationships with others, it's a problem.

ALERT

Anger is a common symptom of a blood sugar low. If you feel yourself getting angry for no good reason, it may be a sign you need to test your blood sugar. And if you live with someone with diabetes, try not to take anger personally when it occurs in connection with a low.

Feeling Guilty

It may not be rational, but it's perfectly normal to feel guilty about having diabetes. But now that you know it's normal, it's time to move on. You are not to blame for having diabetes, nor should you feel ashamed of your diagnosis. You've done nothing to deserve your disease; your genetic makeup and/or environmental factors have made you susceptible to it through no fault of your own.

Managing Stress and Burnout

When you face a physically or psychologically stressful situation, your body starts a complex process of hormone release and reaction. The adrenal glands start to pump out cortisol, the hormone primarily responsible for our physiological "fight or flight" reaction to situations humans perceive as dangerous. Cortisol signals the liver to start up glucose production to give the brain and central nervous system added energy, while signaling the fat and muscle tissues to slow their uptake. At the same time, it causes the release of fatty acids from fat tissues, which are needed for muscle fuel, and sends your blood pressure up.

Stress also prompts the adrenal glands to release epinephrine, the hormone that provides the adrenaline rush of the "fight or flight" reaction. High levels of circulating cortisol and epinephrine promote insulin resistance in addition to ratcheting up blood sugar levels. Since it increases blood pressure and glucose levels, stress is obviously not the best medicine for diabetes control. And it's dangerous because it may distract you from controlling your diabetes as you become preoccupied with other issues.

ESSENTIAL

No one, and that means no one, has perfect diabetes management skills all the time. If you have an unforeseen high or low, don't take it as a sign of personal failure. Measure your success by your commitment to care. When a high or low happens, learn from the experience to prevent it the next time.

The Physical Toll

When you're ill or suffer an injury, your body is stressed and you need to test more frequently. The same goes for times when you are mentally and emotionally under duress. Audited by the IRS? On double shifts at work? Taking final exams? Make sure you test blood sugar levels more often than usual.

There is some evidence that extreme, chronic stress may actually cause or predispose an individual to type 2 diabetes. However, stress has also been associated with abdominal or visceral adiposity (that "apple" shape), so it's unclear whether stress causes a spare tire and the spare tire causes type 2, or if the link is a more direct one.

FACT

Physical stress like injury, illness, or trauma typically causes blood sugar levels to rise in diabetes. The stress hormones epinephrine and cortisol amp up blood sugar production. Psychological, or mental, stress also causes hyperglycemia.

Make a Change

Studies have shown that stress management programs can be extremely effective in improving psychological well-being and diabetes control. One Duke University study published in *Diabetes Care* found that just five sessions of stress management training lowered A1C levels an average of half a percentage point. The Duke study involved a stress-training regimen of audiotape-led progressive muscle relaxation, cognitive and behavioral therapy (including guided imagery and deep-breathing exercises), and education on the mechanisms and health consequences of stress. Other good stress management techniques include meditation, yoga, music or art therapy, and journaling. Anything that calms you and allows you to relax and release is a good stress management strategy.

Turning to a Support Group

Support groups are an absolutely invaluable resource for adults with diabetes. A support group offers patients a chance to compare treatment notes, to talk about emotional issues in living with the disease—even to air their gripes about the health care system. In addition to expanding your knowledge and fostering a sense of camaraderie, a support group is a good stress-release valve.

Your doctor's office and/or local hospital are good places to check on existing support groups. If you find that your community doesn't have one, ask your physician or diabetes educator about the possible interest level in a group among other patients. You may be able to set up one of your own.

Around the World

Online communities for people with diabetes are plentiful and can be almost as—if not more—supportive and informative than real-time groups. There's input from Pennsylvania to Paris, with participants from all walks of life and a broad range of experience with diabetes and diabetic complications. On the other hand, you may get inaccurate medical information from people who either don't know better or are trying to sell some miracle cure. The "miracle" workers can be taken care of with the firm hand of a good community moderator. And as long as you take what you read with a grain of salt, you certainly stand more to gain than you can lose. And the beauty of an online support group is that it is there all day and all night for your questions, vents, and gripes.

The Dating Game

Single with diabetes? You may feel like every encounter is a blind date as you consider whether to "tell" about your diabetes. Or you may screen your potential partners by specifically mentioning the D word. There's no reason to treat your diabetes as a skeleton in the closet or a state secret, but some people feel more comfortable sharing their disease after they've laid the foundation for a relationship. The bottom line is, you should do what feels right to you.

Intimacy Issues

When things get intimate, they can also get a little weird. What if you go low and pass out in the heat of passion? Or what if your partner gets tangled up in your infusion set? Having a sexual encounter of the strange kind is the worst nightmare of many single people living with diabetes.

Making love with a partner you trust can alleviate much of the tension you might feel about your first time together. And what seems mortifying now is usually good for a laugh together later. The worst-case scenario rarely happens. Don't obsess over the "coulds" to the point where they become a major preoccupation.

For Spouses and Significant Others

When your partner is handed a diabetes diagnosis, so are you. Get on board with diabetes care right off the bat. You can and should attend diabetes education classes to learn more about the disease and how to treat it. If you do the grocery shopping and/or cooking in your household, you should absolutely attend the meeting your partner has with a registered dietitian. And if your partner feels comfortable with it, go along on doctor's visits as well. Two sets of ears are always better than one.

Try (and it can be hard) not to become the diabetes police. Think of what it would be like to go through life listening to the following:

- "Are you sure you can eat that?"
- "Do you really think you should have that?"
- "Don't you think you should do something about that blood glucose reading?"

Communicate openly and honestly with your partner about how you can help when things aren't going right, before they go astray. That way you know in advance the most effective way to assist.

ALERT

Support your spouse or partner, but keep in mind that she, and not you, is in charge of taking care of her diabetes. This means being there for her if she asks for help, offering to go to the doctor's appointments with her, but not pushing the issue, and not eating things that she can't have right in front of her.

Helping Those Who Don't Help Themselves

Perhaps you're reading this book because you're more interested in diabetes control than your significant other—the one with the disease—is. Maybe your partner hasn't come to terms with his diagnosis yet, or maybe he's depressed or disheartened and has stopped trying. You can read and learn until you're blue in the face, and you may even be able to nag your partner into a few extra blood sugar checks or a more appropriate meal. But you can't control his diabetes for him. Remember this if you remember nothing else. Your mental health and emotional well-being are just as important as your partner's, and you can save yourself countless hours of head-banging frustration if you detach enough to realize that he is the pilot of the diabetes ship.

QUESTION

My husband has had problems in the bedroom ever since he was diagnosed with type 2 diabetes. Is this part of the disease?
If your husband is newly diagnosed, he may be struggling to come to terms with diabetes. Depression, anxiety, and anger are all common emotions following diagnosis of a chronic illness, and could temporarily affect his libido. However, diabetes-associated impotence is quite common.

At the same time, you don't want to go too far in the other direction and make it easier for your partner to get away with screwing up his control by going along with his program. Accepting his excuses about why that extra piece of pie just had to be eaten or nodding your head when she says skipping her meds is not a big deal is not being supportive. It's called "enabling," and spouses and family members of alcoholics do it all the time. Don't let yourself become part of the problem or validate bad behaviors.

CHAPTER 19

Living Life with Diabetes

In theory, there's nothing you can't do now that you couldn't do before you had diabetes. But in practice, you will have to make some lifestyle adjustments to manage your disease well. It's kind of like that tired old joke about the violin— "Doctor, will I ever be able to play the violin again? Yes? But I couldn't play it before. . . ." You may actually be able to do things bigger and better than you could before your diagnosis.

Disclosure

To tell or not to tell? For a lot of people living with diabetes, this can be a tricky question. Some people feel that diabetes is a part of who they are, and share openly. Others may be self-conscious or embarrassed, and keep it to themselves. Or, your reasons for not sharing may simply be personal privacy.

In some cases, however, letting people know you have type 2 diabetes is in your best personal health interest. If you don't generally like to disclose, consider letting people know under the following circumstances.

- **At school.** For children and adolescents who are living with type 2 diabetes, it's important that the school nurse and other appropriate personnel know about the child's condition. Special accommodations may also be provided if your child needs them.
- **In the gym (or other exercise locations).** If you take insulin or other diabetes drugs that put you at risk for hypoglycemia, it's good to have a friend to exercise with who knows about your condition and can help in case of emergency.
- **At the airport.** If you are traveling with blood sugar testing supplies or insulin, you need to let TSA security personnel know about your diabetes. If you wear an insulin pump, you should not have to disconnect to get through security.
- **When getting medical care.** If you are getting any type of emergency or other medical care from anyone that isn't your regular doctor, always mention your diabetes and the medications you take. Illness and injuries drive up blood sugar levels so it's important that a healthcare provider know this fact.
- **In the workplace.** Work is a whole different world, with its own set of considerations discussed later in this chapter. But generally speaking, if you are at risk for low blood sugars, it's a good idea to let at least some of your coworkers know about your condition so they can help you during a hypoglycemic episode if you need it.

Diabetes at Home

Even though you're the one with the diabetes diagnosis, your whole family needs to make some adjustments to living with the disease. A healthful life-style promoting good blood glucose control is the best defense against diabetic complications. And the good news is that it's a great prescription for everyone around you as well.

Don't try to go it alone. The changes that diabetes brings to the dinner table can be positive ones for the entire family, particularly if your diet before now has been less than stellar. Exercise is also a healthy choice for the whole family, both physically and on a psychological level—the family that plays together stays together. You may hear the "why should we all have to suffer?" defense as you encourage your family to join you on your new and more healthful lifestyle. Step back and assess what might be causing that reaction. Fear of giving up the familiar is one possibility. You might also be asking them to do too much too fast, particularly if you were stuck in a fast-food routine.

Start Out Slowly

Try limiting restaurant food to once a week and encouraging healthier menu choices. Instead of mandating "no junk food" off the bat, allow one selection of their choosing to be kept in a cabinet you don't frequent. Above all, work to provide many healthful, fresh, and good-tasting alternatives so the change is perceived as a positive one.

ALERT

While kids should be able to enjoy the occasional treat that isn't regularly on your meal plan, stocking up on junk food isn't healthy for you or them. You don't need the temptation, and they will be better off with more balanced fare.

If your family members have a favorite food that's a no-no for you, only keep it on hand if you're sure it won't be calling you from the cupboard. Remember, you are not an ogre for requesting that potato chips, Moon Pies, and Lucky Charms be kept out of the pantry. No matter what degree of pouting and resistance you face from your spouse or children, stand firm. Bypassing these treats won't harm their health, but having them could very well hurt yours.

Make Your Needs Known

It's easy to get discouraged and depressed when others don't seem to be meeting your needs or even seem to be aware that you have them. Stop those feelings before they start by laying out exactly what you need from the people around you. If you find you don't have enough time to exercise as you should because of child care responsibilities, tell your spouse it's essential to your health to get some assistance.

If your significant other keeps making you all the things you shouldn't be eating, give her some guidance, go with her on the next grocery shopping expedition, or, better yet, take her with on your next appointment with the CDE or dietitian. Don't expect your family and friends to be mind readers. Assume they know next to nothing about your new lifestyle needs, and educate them accordingly.

ESSENTIAL

Stress is a well-known offender in causing blood sugar levels to rise, particularly in patients with type 2 diabetes. Yoga, progressive relaxation, massage therapy, exercise, and meditation are just a few ways to de-stress. Talk therapy, either one-on-one with a counselor or in a support group, can also be extremely helpful.

Making Your Home Diabetes-Friendly

There's more to treatment success than whipping the pantry into shape. The first is keeping a frequent watch on where your blood sugar levels are. One way to encourage yourself is to have several meters available where you'll use them—in the kitchen, by your bed, in your gym bag. If you're often testing at night, there's at least one model on the market with a glow-in-the-dark faceplate for easier testing.

You can use your kitchen timer or alarm clock to remind you to take any postprandial (after-meal) blood sugar checks. Keep several blood sugar logs with your meters so you remember to record your results, or carry a pocket-sized "master log" with you to keep everything in one place.

Home safety is also an issue. If you don't have one already, get a sharps disposal bin. Even if you don't use insulin, you should still have one for your lancets.

Diabetes at Work

If you are employed outside the home, you may need to make some adjustments in your daily work routine to accommodate good treatment habits. There's probably no job out there that is perfectly suited for diabetes, but there are some employment situations that are more difficult than others. Working a job where you're on your feet all day, where it's difficult to take a break to test your blood sugar, where your shifts are unpredictable, or where you are exposed to extreme heat or cold can make control hard.

You may be faced with some tough choices as you try to make your job compatible with your new life. The legal protections offered by the Americans with Disabilities Act will help to a degree, but even with that, you may find yourself in a position where your job is working against your diabetes management. If this is the case, you do have options:

- Talk to your doctor about adjustments to your treatment. Could a new medication or insulin regimen help?
- Talk to your boss or manager about adjustments to your work schedule or other accommodations. Is a transfer possible or preferred? Could a shift change be in order?
- Explore your options both inside and outside of your company. If you've been contemplating a career change or return to school, maybe now is the time to get moving.

Third-shift work and swing-shift work (where your work shifts are switched on a regular basis) are particularly hard on diabetes management, which requires balance. If you must work these types of hours, you need to stay in close contact with your diabetes care team to keep on top of problems as they arise and make any necessary medication and insulin adjustments.

Discrimination: What the Law Says

The Americans with Disabilities Act, passed in 1992, prevents your employer from discriminating against you solely based on your diabetes, and it requires that employers make "reasonable accommodations" to allow you to check your blood sugar and treat yourself as needed. Under the act, a disability is a record of "physical or mental impairment that substantially limits one or more of the major life activities" of an individual. The ADA applies to all employers with fifteen or more employees.

QUESTION

I don't consider myself disabled just because I have diabetes. Am I sending the wrong message if I claim protection under the ADA?
The ADA was designed to cover a broad range of Americans who may experience discrimination in the workplace due to health issues, and is your best protection for fair treatment on the job. When you invoke your rights under the ADA, you ensure you are judged on your abilities rather than your disease.

Providing a small refrigerator for your supplies, giving you short breaks to check your blood sugar, and adjusting your work shift if it causes control problems would all fall under the scope of reasonable accommodation in most cases. If the accommodation is said to provide "undue hardship" on the employer (usually in terms of financial resources), it may not be required. Generally speaking, the majority of accommodations that would be required for diabetes would not be considered an undue hardship under the ADA for most organizations. However, you should consult a lawyer specializing in disability law if you have specific questions about your situation and employer.

Your employer cannot deny you health benefits; under the ADA, you are entitled to the same health insurance, disability, and other benefits as other employees in your workplace. And if your spouse or child develops diabetes and you carry insurance for your family through your employer, you are covered by these same provisions.

Job Hunting

Looking for a job? The ADA protects you against discrimination here as well. Know that questions about your health in an interview are illegal, and so is withdrawing a job offer based on your diabetes alone. If your diabetes is disclosed during a pre-employment physical, your prospective employer cannot use it as a reason to deny you employment as long as reasonable accommodations can be made for you. Of course, going for the head wine-taster job at the local vineyard may not be a good idea; there may be certain positions that require activities you just can't perform or that can't be "reasonably accommodated."

ALERT

If, based on the employer's words or actions, you have any reason to believe you were discriminated against because of your disease, contact the Equal Employment Opportunity Commission at 1-800-669-4000. There are time limits for filing discrimination claims (180 to 300 days depending on the circumstances), so contact the EEOC as soon as possible to determine if you have a legitimate claim.

In addition, you may be legally unable to obtain licensure for certain positions like commercial truck driving, depending on the state you live in. However, if you already work one of these positions and develop diabetes, your employer must offer you another suitable vacant position within the company (as long as you are qualified to perform the new job). The ADA also prevents your employer from denying you a promotion based on your diabetes.

Workplace Accommodations

There are many benefits to providing a working environment that accommodates people with diabetes and other chronic illnesses. Employee satisfaction, better retention rate, fewer sick days, and lower disability pay-out are just a few good motivations. It also takes money and resources to train employees, and if you are a good worker, it makes sense for your employer to do what it can to retain you.

If the people in your workplace don't seem to know a lot about diabetes, take the opportunity to teach them. Let your human resources director know about the Diabetes at Work program (*www.diabetesatwork.org*), which educates employers about diabetes and offers advice on instituting screening and wellness programs designed to reduce diabetic complications. The American Diabetes Association is also an excellent source of information for your employer.

FACT

Under the ADA, your employer must maintain your confidentiality about your health condition, disclosing it to others only on a "need to know" basis (for example, if you work in a manufacturing environment where a company nurse is on staff, she would be informed of your condition so she could treat you appropriately).

To Tell or Not to Tell

Telling others can be hard. You may be afraid of job discrimination. And sometimes it can be difficult admitting you need help. However, you can't claim protection under the ADA if you don't let your employer know about your condition and ask for accommodation assistance. If you're inexplicably missing work or taking longer or more frequent breaks without permission, you may very well lose your job.

There are several good reasons to let your coworkers in on your diabetes. First, people around you need to know what to do in case of a blood sugar emergency. Second, it's an excellent opportunity to spread awareness of the disease and perhaps educate coworkers in the process. And finally, if your employer has allowed you extra breaks and other accommodations to check your blood sugar levels and treat yourself, letting coworkers in on the reason can prevent feelings of ill will.

Eat, Drink, and Be Wary

Birthday parties, family reunions, wedding receptions, holiday office gatherings—any event where food and drink play a starring role is a potential danger zone without the right preparation. If you know the fare will be high in carbs, bring along a healthy dish (your hostess will probably appreciate the contribution). Having a small snack at home before the event can help to blunt your appetite against too many temptations.

Don't forget that dancing is exercise. Check your blood sugar levels if you've been out on the dance floor for a while to ensure they aren't dropping too low. If food won't be available at all times during the party, bring a snack with you to fuel up. A nondiet soda or juice from the bar can help to treat a low if you're caught without glucose tablets. If you decide to enjoy beer, wine, or a mixed drink, use caution and make sure you have a friend with you who can recognize the signs of a low and treat them accordingly.

Behind the Wheel

Always test before you drive, and if you're low, don't drive. Blood glucose levels below 70 mg/dl should be treated appropriately, and a safe blood sugar level should be attained before getting back behind the wheel. If you start to experience symptoms of hypoglycemia while you are driving, pull over immediately to test and treat. A low impairs your judgment and can cause you to lose consciousness. Like alcohol and falling asleep at the wheel, low blood sugars can easily result in a traffic fatality.

Licensing Issues

For people with well-controlled diabetes and a good driving record, maintaining a noncommercial driver's license shouldn't be an issue. State law governs regulations for driver's licenses, and in some cases your license may have medical restrictions (particularly if you are on insulin). In addition, if you take insulin for your diabetes, you may have your license suspended if you have a history of severe hypoglycemic episodes. In many states, your doctor is required to report you to the department of motor vehicles if he feels it is unsafe for you to drive due to your diabetes. If your diabetes is not well controlled, if you experience hypoglycemic unawareness, if you have frequent lows, or if you have diabetic complications that affect your vision or reaction time, it may not be safe for you to drive a motor vehicle.

Commercial licenses (CDLs) generally have much stricter regulations, again governed by state. In many states, taking insulin is grounds to have your commercial license revoked or not issued. The ADA has been active in advocating the creation of a system that evaluates CDL applications on a case-by-case basis instead of with a blanket ban, and in 2003 legislation that allows for exemption of insulin-taking CDLs who meet specific criteria was passed. Your state motor vehicle bureau can answer specific questions about the licensing laws in your area and how they apply to intrastate commercial driving as well.

FACT

In the mid-1990s, the Federal Aviation Administration overturned a blanket ban on small-aircraft private pilot licenses for people who take insulin for their diabetes. These license applications are now handled on a case-by-case basis, evaluating each individual's specific medical situation rather than discriminating against everyone.

On a Road Trip

The minivan, the open road, passing cornfields, roadside diners, and the hourly "are we there yet?" question. Ahhh—the pleasures of the family road trip. Taking a trip by car brings its own unique set of challenges to people living with diabetes. Prolonged sitting, road fatigue, truck stop dining, and should-have-turned-left-at-the-last-exit-but-won't-ask-for-directions syndrome are just a few of the roadblocks you may have to overcome.

Stop and stretch often to get your circulation going and cut fatigue. It's a good idea to check your blood sugar levels at each rest stop as well. Again, pack snacks just in case you get waylaid, and don't count on the next restaurant being quite so far. A cooler is an excellent idea if you'll be traveling long stretches of remote highways. A cell phone is also essential for rural travel in case a breakdown leaves you stranded or you have a medical emergency. And keep a phone car charger handy, as a dead cell phone won't be of much use to you.

Make sure all insulin, testing kits, and medications are stored in a place that won't get excessively hot or cold. Trunks, glove compartments, and dashboards are all bad spots to keep your supplies. If you're traveling in hot weather and you stop for a food or road break, do not leave your supplies and/or medication in the car unless you have a cooler to store them in. On a 73°F day, in just ten minutes temperatures can reach 100°F and higher in a car with the windows rolled up, which is bound to make your insulin go bad and possibly damage your meter and other equipment.

Be Prepared

Whether you're going by plane, train, or automobile, there are some basics you should carry along with your toothbrush and clean underwear. These include the following:

- A first-aid kit, including antibiotic ointment and bandages
- Extra medication and insulin (and pump supplies, if applicable)
- Blood sugar meter with an ample supply of test strips, alcohol swabs, and lancets
- Extra batteries for your meter
- Emergency supply of fast-acting glucose
- Plenty of snacks, including fast-acting carbs

Always travel with twice the amount of medication and/or insulin you would normally require for the time you'll be gone. The same goes for blood sugar testing supplies. If you are delayed for weather or any other unexpected reason, your foresight will save you a lot of scrambling about trying to get a prescription filled in an unfamiliar place.

A sturdy, watertight supply case is a must for anyone who travels frequently. For those who take insulin, a case that is well padded and insulated to keep vials or pens at their proper temperature is also important. Finally, remember that your supplies should always be transported as carry-on bags versus checked luggage to avoid any problems with lost bags and missing meters and medications.

Travel Tips for the Wise

Vacations and business travel can present some unique control challenges and safety issues. Don't travel completely alone unless you have to. In case of an emergency, a trusted friend, spouse, or companion will be invaluable, particularly if you're in a foreign country. If you're a free spirit and like to fly solo, make sure you always carry your basic medical information (i.e., name, diagnosis, medication, physician contact) on your person, and wear your medical ID.

Air Travel and Medical Devices

In the past few years, air travel security measures have changed significantly in the United States and abroad. Because having diabetes necessitates traveling with medical sharps, there are some extra steps you may need to take to ensure you have easy access to your insulin and testing supplies while flying.

- **Insulin.** Keep all original packaging and paperwork that come with your insulin so you can present the original printed pharmaceutical label for the medication at the airport security checkpoint. The same applies for glucagon kits. Syringes will be allowed past security only if the accompanying medication is properly labeled.
- **Meters.** The FAA will allow glucose meters and lancets in suitcases or carry-on baggage as long as meters are clearly marked with the manufacturer and/or brand name. Lancets should be capped and properly stored with the meter.
- **Pumps and CGMS.** If you wear an insulin pump or continuous monitor, inform airport security personnel and request that they visually inspect it rather than removing it. Several insulin pump manufacturers recommend that you do not go through the full-body scanners while the pump is attached, as the scanner can damage the pump's sensitive electronics. Ask a TSA agent for a pat-down instead. Again, have insulin documentation with you. If screeners insist you remove your insulin pump or walk through a scanner with it on, ask to speak with a security checkpoint supervisor.

Allow plenty of extra time for getting through airport security. You may want to plan on an extra thirty to sixty minutes in addition to whatever your airline is advising for advance arrival time. This will give you breathing room if airport personnel need to check out your medical supplies. And always call the airline you'll be traveling with first to find out its specific security policies for the flight.

ESSENTIAL

A number of diabetes drugs may cause photosensitivity (skin's oversensitivity to the sun). To minimize your risk, wear a brimmed hat and sunscreen with an SPF of 15 or higher for all exposed skin (30 or higher if you have sensitive skin). Long sleeves and pants also increase protection.

If you have problems with improper treatment or discrimination when traveling by air, call the Transportation Security Administration (TSA) Cares hot line at 1-855-787-2227. Complaints may be filed in writing with the Transportation Security Administration, Office of Civil Rights and Liberties (TSA-6), External Compliance Division, 601 South 12th Street, Arlington, VA 20598.

Adjusting Insulin and Time Zones

International travel requires some extra planning, particularly if you take insulin. In addition to the usual jet lag, you have to keep on schedule with your medication. In general, the easiest and most practical approach is to take insulin on track with meals in the "new" time zone you're traveling in (or are en route to). However, you should always consult your doctor or diabetes educator about appropriate adjustments to insulin and medication before you travel, as her advice may vary based on the type of insulin you take, the distance you are traveling, and other factors specific to your situation.

Staying Well Abroad

To safeguard your health and safety while traveling in a foreign country, you should make sure you can communicate your needs adequately and are well supplied for the journey. Some tips:

- **Get your shots.** Before you go, make sure any required immunizations are up-to-date.
- **Learn the language.** If you don't speak the native tongue, make sure you have a guidebook to help you with basic medical phrases like "I need a doctor" and "I have diabetes."
- **Have your papers in order.** Keep your doctor's name and phone number along with your written insulin schedule on you at all times, and, as always, wear your medical identification.
- **Drink water.** If the water is questionable, drink bottled (and hold the ice in any canned and bottled beverages you order) to avoid diarrhea or more serious illnesses.
- **Keep a food supply.** Make sure you have a stash of nonperishable snacks like peanut butter and crackers, canned fruit juice, raisins, dried apricots, nutrition bars, and other foods that keep well and will serve as a mini-meal should your plans be interrupted.
- **Bring plenty of diabetes supplies.** Pack at least two to three times the amount of medication and supplies you will likely need on the trip. A travel delay in a country where you can't get your usual medications and supplies could be catastrophic.

CHAPTER 20

The Future of Type 2 Treatment

Diabetes is, at present, an incurable disease. Although type 2 diabetes can be well controlled to the point of normal or near-normal blood glucose levels, once you have it, it's a lifelong companion. One day advances in medical research may make a cure a reality. But in the meantime, new developments in diabetes drugs and device technology can improve the diabetes health and quality of life for millions of Americans living with the disease.

The "Cure" Word

Although you may see many diet plans, supplement products, and other treatments that claim to "reverse" or "cure" type 2 diabetes, the fact is that there is presently no cure for this chronic, genetically based and environmentally triggered condition. Once you have type 2 diabetes, you will always have type 2 diabetes.

Some treatments can and do control symptoms of the disease, allowing you to live with normal or near normal blood sugar levels for an extended period of time. For example, studies have shown that for some obese patients, successful gastric banding surgery will virtually normalize blood sugar levels. And sometimes, when a young overweight patient loses a considerable amount of weight, the same thing may happen. This "well controlled" type 2 diabetes, where symptoms are in remission, is certainly a great achievement and what all people with type 2 strive toward.

However, diabetes is always there, watching and waiting. And without continued healthy lifestyle habits, including good dietary and carbohydrate management and regular exercise, the symptoms of high blood sugar will return. So a constant vigilance, and an understanding that there is no magic pill or procedure, is important.

Clinical Trials

Clinical trials are scientific research studies that examine different aspects of a disease or medical condition or evaluate new drugs and other treatments. By participating in a clinical trial, you can get free access to new therapies not yet available to others. However, you also take any risks associated with an unproven treatment.

All clinical trials have to meet guidelines outlined by both the National Institutes of Health (NIH) and the U.S. Food and Drug Administration (FDA). They also must meet the specific criteria of the institution that sponsors the research. A governing body known as an institutional review board (IRB) oversees the study design and protocols to ensure it meets specific ethical, clinical, and safety standards.

Clinical trials of new drugs fall into four different "phase" categories. Phase 1 studies are initial, small-scale trials that help establish a safe dose and determine side effects. Phase 2 uses a larger study population at the dose established in phase 1 to determine the efficacy of the drug, and phase 3 studies compare the new drug with existing treatments for the same condition or illness and monitor for side effects. Finally, phase 4 trials are performed after the product is approved and introduced to the marketplace to gather "postmarket" data on its long-term safety and efficacy.

Informed Consent

It's important to note that when you agree to participate in a clinical trial, you may not necessarily receive the treatment that the study is evaluating. Depending on the design of the study, you may be chosen to be part of a control group (members of which do not receive the therapy being tested in order to serve as a baseline for comparison), or you may receive a placebo (an inactive substance that is sometimes administered to half of the study group to measure the effectiveness of the treatment against a control).

QUESTION

How can I find out more about taking part in a clinical trial?
If you're interested in participating in a clinical trial, your first step is to check and see what is available. The government website *www .clinicaltrials.gov* has a database of NIH-sponsored trials. If you live near a research institution or university, you can also check on available clinical trials there. Eligibility requirements will vary with each study.

Learning all of the potential ins and outs of a clinical trial is part of giving informed consent on the study. Because the treatments examined in clinical trials are still experimental, informed consent is an important aspect of meeting the ethical guidelines of scientific study.

Genetic Keys

Type 2 diabetes has a strong genetic link and scientists are discovering new genetic clues each year. As of mid-2012, research had identified nearly forty gene variants that either raise or lower the risk of developing type 2 diabetes.

While genetic risk and variants is influenced by ethnicity, and it's likely that many genes are associated with increased diabetes risk, there is one gene variant at this time that appears to be associated with the highest risk of developing type 2 diabetes across many ethnic groups—the TCF7L2 gene. There is now a blood test for this gene, called deCODE T2 (deCODE Genetics). The test must be ordered by your doctor and may or may not be reimbursable by your health care insurer. Of course, knowing if you have this gene or not does not change the fact that healthy lifestyle changes in diet and exercise patterns, plus maintaining a healthy body weight, are the best way to prevent type 2 diabetes

So why are genetics important to research if you can't do anything to change your DNA? Understanding the genetic causes of type 2 diabetes does two things. First of all, it can help researchers understand how the disease may be prevented in future generations by targeting individuals at risk for early intervention. And secondly, having a clearer picture of the genetic basis of the disease provides scientists with more information to target future diabetes drug development.

Better Drugs

New drugs can take decades to discover and develop, and billions of dollars to bring to market. And while hundreds of diabetes drugs are in development at any given time, only a small fraction of these end up making it all the way through phase 3 clinical trials successfully and are submitted to the FDA for evaluation and approval. A fraction of those are then approved and make it to market. This rigorous process ensures that new prescription drugs are well-tested for safety, but it can also mean a long wait for new medication options for patients.

FACT

Of 101 new drug applications submitted for brand new drug compounds in 2011, the FDA approved 30. Just one of these approved drugs was a diabetes drug. And 2011 was a banner year, the highest since 2004, when the FDA granted 36 total approvals.

As of mid-2012, several new GLP-1 agonists and DPP-4 inhibitor drugs are in late stage development and, pending FDA approval, these drugs will provide even more options for people with type 2. Perhaps more importantly, there are several brand new classes of type 2 diabetes drugs in development that work on unique pathways of the body.

Sodium-Glucose Cotransporter-2 Inhibitors (SGLT2)

One exciting new class of drugs for type 2 diabetes is the sodium-glucose cotransporter-2 inhibitors (SGLT2). This class of drugs targets the kidneys and lowers blood sugar by causing more glucose to leave the body through the urine. In clinical trials, SGLT2 drugs have shown an added clinical benefit—weight loss.

The first drug of this class submitted for approval in the United States was Forxiga (dapagliflozin). But in early 2012, the U.S. Food and Drug Administration asked drug developers Bristol-Myers Squibb Co. and AstraZeneca to submit more clinical data before they would consider approval of the drug. In trials, the drug was associated with some bladder and breast cancers and liver problems in a small percentage of patients. As of mid-2012, the two companies were still conducting trials of the drug to gather the requested data.

A second SGLT2 drug, canagliflozin (from Jannsen, a division of Johnson and Johnson), was submitted to the FDA in June of 2012. Several other drug manufacturers have their own SGLT2 drugs in the pipeline. This drug class is expected to be an important new tool for millions of Americans living with type 2 diabetes.

GPR40 Agonists

GPR40 agonists differ from other drug classes in that they only stimulate insulin secretion when high blood sugar levels are present. The first drug in this class to reach phase 3 clinical trials, TAK-875 (from Takeda), has demonstrated good clinical results. A three-month trial found the drug brought A1C levels down an average of 1 percentage point with few side effects. The big advantage of the drug seems to be that it does not cause hypoglycemia.

New Insulins

Several innovative new insulin products are in the drug development pipeline. The first, Afrezza, would be the only inhalable insulin on the U.S. market if approved by the FDA. The second, Tresiba, would provide type 2 patients with an ultra–long acting, peakless basal insulin that lasts longer than any currently available insulin product.

Afrezza is an ultra–rapid acting insulin that is inhaled instead of injected. The insulin comes in a fine powder formulation, which is delivered via a small inhaler, not unlike an asthma inhaler. In clinical trials, Afrezza demonstrated a lower risk of hypoglycemia and of insulin-related weight gain than its noninhalable counterparts. And of course, an insulin that is inhaled instead of injected may be a better alternative for a needle-shy patient who is just starting on insulin.

In 2010, the FDA asked MannKind, the drug manufacturer of Afrezza, to provide more extensive clinical data before it would move forward in consideration of approving Afrezza. As of the writing of this book, additional clinical trials were taking place. If Afrezza is approved, it will actually become the second inhalable insulin to make it to the U.S. market. The first inhaled insulin, Exubera (Pfizer), was withdrawn by the manufacturer due to lackluster sales.

Other new insulins that don't require injection are also in development. Oral-lyn (Generex) is a spray insulin that is administered to the buccal membrane, or inside of the cheek, via an inhaler device. The drug manufacturer, Generex, is currently designing phase 3 trials for the drug.

Tresiba (degludec), the first ultra–long acting basal insulin analog, was submitted for FDA approval by manufacturer Novo Nordisk in 2011. Tresiba has a duration of action of over forty hours, making it the longest acting basal insulin yet. In clinical trials, the new insulin demonstrated a lower incidence of low blood sugar episodes than currently available basal insulin products. An FDA decision on Tresiba is expected in late 2012.

Better Devices

Improvements in blood sugar monitoring technology can also make a big difference in your diabetes health and quality of life. These improved devices that provide patients with more convenience, more information, and less discomfort show great promise for people living with type 2 diabetes.

Noninvasive Blood Sugar Testing Technologies

Blood sugar monitoring that doesn't involve actually drawing blood is the holy grail of diabetes devices. There are other noninvasive options in development that could eliminate the blood draw. A device called Easy Check (from PositiveID) is a breathalyzer-type device that checks glucose levels by measuring the amount of acetone in exhaled air. The patient breathes into the device, and the exhaled air is mixed with a chemical compound within the unit. The results are then measured, put through a mathematical algorithm, and translated into a standard mg/dl blood sugar measurement on the device's display unit. The company began human clinical trials of the product in early 2012.

QUESTION

I saw on the news that there is a blood sugar tattoo that reads your levels. Where can I get one of those?
Researchers at several institutions are developing blood glucose "tattoos" that use nanotechnology to monitor and display blood sugar levels. The tattoo "ink" contains nanoparticles that are injected into the skin and can detect current blood sugar levels when a second external device is held or worn over the tattoo. The technology is still in its very early stages and it will likely be years before it is available to most people with type 2.

Other technologies under development for both blood sugar testing and continuous glucose monitoring that don't involve lancing the skin include infrared, spectroscopy, and even contact lenses that measure the glucose in tears. These and other new monitoring technologies that reduce patient discomfort and cost may help to increase testing compliance.

Noninvasive Continuous Glucose Monitoring

While continuous glucose monitoring (CGM) systems are a great step forward in monitoring blood sugar trends, they still require regular finger sticks to calibrate and a sensor and needle insertion into the skin. One device currently in clinical trials, the Symphony tCGM system (from Echo Therapeutics), uses a needleless transdermal (through the skin) system that measures glucose levels in interstitial fluid. The Symphony then transmits the glucose readings wirelessly every minute to a remote device or smartphone. Preliminary trials have found the device to be highly accurate in both type 1 and type 2 diabetes patients.

Building a Better Pancreas

One goal of current diabetes research is to find a way to "close the loop" on glucose monitoring and insulin treatment. This means creating a device that will monitor blood sugar levels and deliver the correct amount of insulin in response without any required operator intervention. Basically, this device would act as an electronic artificial pancreas. While the artificial pancreas would primarily benefit people with type 1 diabetes, it may one day also be a valuable treatment tool for those with type 2 diabetes as well.

Half of this technology already exists in the continuous glucose monitoring (CGM) systems that have hit the market in recent years. The trick is to get the CGM system to do some complex calculations that translate current blood sugar readings into an accurate insulin dose, and then relay the dosage information to an insulin pump to carry out delivery. Unfortunately, many of today's CGM systems still have a wide margin of accuracy error, so further refinement of the technology and the mathematical algorithms that program it must be done before CGM is ready for closed-loop prime time.

In 2012, medical device manufacturer Medtronic filed an application with the FDA to approve the Paradigm Veo pump, an insulin pump and integrated CGM device. The Veo is the first pump that features an automatic shutoff for insulin flow once it detects that blood sugar levels have fallen below a set point. The device is already approved and in use in fifty other countries.

As of mid-2012, several small trials have shown successful results with artificial pancreas technology. Larger trials with more patients trying these devices under "real world" conditions will be needed to test and refine the treatment and prove its long-term value.

Advocacy Groups

You literally have the power of millions on your side in the fight against diabetes. Along with the nearly 26 million Americans living with this disease, high-clout national advocacy organizations like the American Diabetes Association fight each day for diabetes rights, treatment advances, and a permanent solution to the disease—a cure.

Diabetes research also has many friends on Capitol Hill, including senators and representatives who have personally been touched by the disease. By adding your voice to the call for increases in research funding, both through your vote and with your support of advocacy and education in your community, you take the cause a little bit further. Yes, diabetes is a powerful enemy, but with strength in numbers, the fight can be won.

Additional Resources

General Diabetes Information

dLife—For Your Diabetes Life
This site offers the largest collection of diabetes videos on the web that run the gamut from cooking to celebrity profiles to diabetes "how tos."
www.dlife.com

Taking Care of Your Diabetes
Established by endocrinologist Dr. Steve Edelman, this unique series of national conferences offers people with diabetes a day of education and connection with others. You can find a conference near you on their website, or learn from some of their many videos and features online.
www.tcoyd.org

Joslin Diabetes Center
The world-renowned Boston-based Joslin Diabetes Center is a leading diabetes care and research facility. They also have accredited satellite programs throughout the United States and fantastic online resources.
www.joslin.org

National Diabetes Education Program (NDEP)
The NDEP helps translate the latest diabetes research into practical information for people with diabetes. Their website features many free, downloadable publications.
ndep.nih.gov

National Institute of Diabetes and Digestive and Kidney Diseases (NIDDK)
One of the National Institutes of Health, this government organization offers information on diabetes, weight control, diabetic kidney disease, and more.
www.niddk.nih.gov

Food and Nutrition

Academy of Nutrition and Dietetics
Formerly the American Dietetic Association, the Academy of Nutrition and Dietetics is the national organization for all registered dietitians in the United States.
www.eatright.org

dLife Recipe Finder

Search thousands of recipes by course and carb level. Each one has full nutritional analysis.

www.dLife.com/recipebox

University of Sydney's Glycemic Index

This internationally recognized center of nutritional research offers a full searchable database of GI and GL values.

www.glycemicindex.com

Fitness and Exercise

Dance Out Diabetes

A San Francisco–based organization with a mission to "prevent and manage diabetes through dance, education, support and increased access to care."

www.danceoutdiabetes.org

American Council of Exercise (ACE)

A nonprofit organization that certifies fitness professionals and promotes safe and effective physical activity. The ACE GetFit consumer area of their website offers an entire section on exercising with type 2 diabetes.

www.acefitness.org/fitfacts

Type 2 Diabetes Patient Blogs

Blogabetes

People from all parts of the diabetes community share their stories and challenges on this dLife blog.

www.dlife.com/diabetes-blog

Living with Diabetes

One of the longest running diabetes blogs on the web, and authored by type 2 teacher and dog lover Kathleen Weaver.

www.kweaver.us/blog

Kids and Teens with Diabetes

Children with Diabetes

The award-winning Children with Diabetes site features a special dedicated forum area for parents of children with type 2 diabetes to ask questions and get support.

forums.childrenwithdiabetes.com

Diabetes Education and Camping Association (DECA)

Camp is a great way for children to learn more about caring for their condition, meet others like them, and have fun doing it. Many camps now offer type 2 programs for kids. Search DECA's extensive database for a camp near you.

www.diabetescamps.org

Living with My Type 2

This site was created to support a PBS special on teens and type 2. It features compelling video diaries from teens.

www.pbs.org/mytype2

Finding Your Health Care Team

American Association of Clinical Endocrinologists (AACE)

Endocrinologists are physicians that have specialized expertise in diseases of the endocrine system, such as diabetes. The AACE website allows you to search for an endocrinologist in your area who specializes in diabetes care.

www.aace.com

American Association of Diabetes Educators (AADE)

Diabetes education is a cornerstone of good diabetes control. The AADE can help you locate an educator near you.

800-338-3633

www.diabeteseducator.org

American Academy of Dermatology (AAD)

Search for a dermatologist in your area to treat diabetic skin conditions.

www.aad.org

American Academy of Neurology (AAN)

If you suffer from neuropathy, you may need to see a neurologist. The AAN has a searchable database of board certified neurologists at their patient website.

800-879-1960

patients.aan.com

American Academy of Ophthalmology (AAO)

People with diabetes need a dilated eye exam at least once a year. If you don't have a regular ophthalmologist, the AAO can help you locate an eye doctor near you.

www.aao.org

American Podiatric Medical Association (APMA)

Good foot care is imperative to people with diabetes. The APMA can connect you to a podiatrist in your area, as well as providing helpful expert information to treat feet right.

800-ASK-APMA

www.apma.org

Pediatric Endocrine Society (PES)

Find a pediatric endocrinologist in the PES searchable database.

703-556-9222

www.lwpes.org

Travel with Diabetes

CDC Travelers' Health
Get the health basics on overseas destinations.
www.cdc.gov/travel

Society for Accessible Travel and Hospitality (SATH)
Planning a trip? SATH can help you find some diabetes-friendly accommodations for your journey.
www.sath.org

Transportation Security Administration (TSA)
Check out the latest security guidelines and precautions for travelers with diabetes before you fly.
www.tsa.gov/travelers/airtravel/specialneeds/index.shtm

Advocacy Organizations

American Diabetes Association (ADA)
The ADA sets clinical diabetes standards for U.S. physicians and also acts on behalf of diabetes patients to fund research and fight discrimination.
1-800-DIABETES
www.diabetes.org

Canadian Diabetes Association (CDA)
The CDA is "leading the fight against diabetes by helping people with diabetes live healthy lives while working to find the cure."
www.diabetes.ca

Diabetes Hands Foundation
Established by TuDiabetes founder Manny Hernandez, this nonprofit organization is dedicated to connecting, engaging, and empowering people touched by diabetes.
www.diabeteshandsfoundation.org

International Diabetes Federation (IDF)

The IDF is an umbrella organization of over 200 national diabetes associations, such as the ADA, in over 160 countries. The organization promotes World Diabetes Day on November 14 each year.

www.idf.org

Patient Assistance Programs

The Partnership for Prescription Assistance (PPA)

If you are uninsured or underinsured, a patient assistance program may help you get needed diabetes drugs for little to no cost. Call or visit the website to find out if you are eligible.

1-888-4PPA-NOW

www.pparx.org

Support Groups and Communities

American Diabetes Association

A robust forum-based community, moderated by ADA staff and volunteers.

community.diabetes.org

Dear Janis, with CDE/RD Janis Roszler

Certified diabetes educator, marriage and family therapist, and registered dietitian Janis Roszler oversees this excellent site that features a small but active diabetes forum.

www.dearjanis.com

Diabetes Daily

A community-focused site featuring blogs, groups, chats, and online workshops. Run by Elizabeth and David Edelman.

www.diabetesdaily.com

Diabetes Sisters

Diabetes activist Brandy Barnes launched this diabetes community in 2008 as a safe place for women to talk about the unique diabetes issues they face. In addition to the online community forums, you can find a local or national meeting, sign up for the mentoring "Sister Match" program, or read some of the featured blogs and expert commentary.

www.diabetessisters.org

Divabetic

Geared toward women but open to all, this grassroots organization was founded by Max Szadak. Max was an assistant to singer Luther Vandross, who passed away from type 2 diabetes–related complications in 2005. Divabetic strives to make the process of learning about diabetes self-management fun and enjoyable.

www.divabetic.org

TuDiabetes

Run by the Diabetes Hands Foundation, this vibrant community site offers lively discussion, blogs, groups, videos, and special promotions.

www.tudiabetes.com

APPENDIX B

Preventive Care Guidelines

Regular preventive care is especially important when you have diabetes. The following chart is based on the recommended preventive care testing guidelines from both the American Diabetes Association and the American Association of Clinical Endocrinologists. **Please remember that these are guidelines only, and you may need more frequent and/or additional diagnostic testing based on your particular medical history and diabetic complications.** For example, if you have known kidney problems, your physician will test your microalbumin levels more frequently, and if you have coronary artery disease, your regular visits may include additional cardiovascular assessment. Your diabetes care provider should discuss testing recommendations specific to your needs.

	Quarterly Exams	Annual Exams	Each Office Visit
Blood pressure and pulse			X
Height and weight			X
*Cholesterol (lipid panel)		X	
Comprehensive dilated-eye exam		X	
Foot exam			X
A1C**	X		
Microalbumin		X	
Serum creatinine		X	

*Most adult patients should have fasting lipid profiles performed at least annually, according to ADA guidelines. Low-risk adults (LDL <100 mg/dl, HDL >50 mg/dl, triglycerides <150) can be tested every two years.

**If patient is at A1C goal and is stable, the A1C may be performed twice a year.

Sources: ADA Standards of Medical Care for Patients with Diabetes Mellitus, Diabetes Care, 2012; AACE Diabetes Care Plan Guidelines, 2011.

Index

We Have EVERYTHING® on Anything!

With more than 19 million copies sold, the Everything® series has become one of America's favorite resources for solving problems, learning new skills, and organizing lives. Our brand is not only recognizable—it's also welcomed.

The series is a hand-in-hand partner for people who are ready to tackle new subjects—like you!

For more information on the Everything® series, please visit *www.adamsmedia.com*

The Everything® list spans a wide range of subjects, with more than 500 titles covering 25 different categories:

Business	History	Reference
Careers	Home Improvement	Religion
Children's Storybooks	Everything Kids	Self-Help
Computers	Languages	Sports & Fitness
Cooking	Music	Travel
Crafts and Hobbies	New Age	Wedding
Education/Schools	Parenting	Writing
Games and Puzzles	Personal Finance	
Health	Pets	